GETTING HEALTHY

50 Lessons on Fitness for Law Enforcement

Matthew Wagner, Ph.D.
Joe Serio, Ph.D.

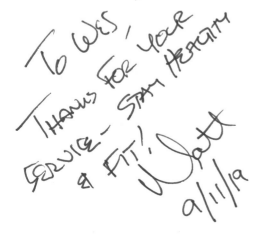

To Wes,
Thanks for your
service - stay Healthy
& fit! [signature]
2/11/19

Project Manager: Jennifer Serio
Design Team: Harriet McHale and Tracey Neikirk

Printed in the United States of America
ISBN 13: 978-0-9900216-5-0

www.LEDtraining.com

Contents

The long span of the bridge of your life is supported by countless cables called habits, attitudes, and desires. What you do in life depends upon what you are and what you want. What you get from life depends upon how much you want it, how much you are willing to work and plan and cooperate and use your resources. The long span of the bridge of your life is supported by countless cables that you are spinning now, and that is why today is such an important day. Make the cables strong!

~ L.G. Elliott

Titles in the
Law Enforcement Development Series

Dispatcher Stress: 50 Lessons on Beating the Burnout

Leaving Blue: 50 Lessons on Retiring Well from Law Enforcement – Financial Aspects

Leaving Blue: 50 Lessons on Retiring Well from Law Enforcement – Emotional Aspects

For more information about these titles in this series, please visit us at www.LEDtraining.com

Introduction

*For, usually and fitly, the presence of an introduction
is held to imply that there is something of
consequence and importance to be introduced.*

~ Arthur Machen

You know what you need to do. You've spent a long time ignoring what you need to do. And guess what? The problem remains.

You've probably heard the popularized definition of insanity: doing the same thing over and over and expecting a different result. That applies to everything in your life, including exercise, health, and fitness. If you don't change something, nothing will change. Guaranteed.

Unfortunately, law enforcement is less fit in most areas than at least half of all U.S. citizens despite the fact that the physical demands of the job require that you be more fit than the average person.

As a group, your fitness levels are below normal in the areas of aerobic fitness, body fat, and abdominal strength. In upper body strength and lower-back flexibility, you were found to be just average, according to a study conducted from 1983 to 1993 by the Cooper Institute for Aerobics Research.

Law enforcement officers have a greater morbidity and mortality rate than the general public, due mostly to cardiovascular disease, colon cancer, and suicide.

The risk of having a heart attack doubles with each decade of law enforcement service.

In 2014, Harvard School of Public Health and the Cambridge Health Alliance discovered that police officers in the U.S. face roughly a 30 to 70 times higher risk of Sudden Cardiac Death (SCD) when you're involved in stressful situations vs. routine non-stressful situations. Part of the problem is so many of your situations are stressful.

Unfortunately, for many of you, serious attention to fitness and health ended shortly after you left the academy.

You may be overweight or feel sluggish. You may have ailments such as diabetes and take a handful of prescription medications on a daily basis. You may be achy and generally miserable most of the time.

The good news is you can turn this around. Through simple activity and exercise routines, you don't have to become a statistic.

Exercise, fitness, and health will dramatically improve your attitude, relationships, performance, and satisfaction.

Exercise, fitness, and health will greatly reduce your need for medication, will improve the way you feel, and will help make your career and your retirement a much more positive experience.

Exercise, fitness, and health are the foundation that makes everything else possible. Without it, you're limited in what you can do for your department, your community, your family, or yourself.

This book is a simple prescription for law enforcement officers who need to get moving. It's a first step in your transformation to having the life and health you want.

If you already workout on a regular basis, stay active, watch your weight, eat right, and have few physical issues, this book is not for you. If you have no problem being motivated to exercise and lose weight, this book isn't for you.

How to Use This Book

Getting Healthy: 50 Lessons on Fitness for Law Enforcement is a practical guide to help you get past any fear and procrastination surrounding exercise and help you take steps to improve your life.

This book is arranged in eight parts.

Part 1, Exercise Fitness and Health, provides a brief overview of exercise, fitness, and health, and makes the very important distinction between exercise and activity.

Part 2, Facing Fear, is the core of the psychological aspect of exercising. The biggest obstacle we have in our lives is knowing how to win the head game, and getting out to exercise is mostly a head game.

Part 3, Creating a System, is the critical section in the book. Without a system in place to go get what you want, the odds are very high that you won't. This part shows you how to set yourself up for success.

Part 4, Components of Fitness, presents the foundations of the exercise part of the book. It helps you start to get more specific about what you need to do and how you need to do it.

Part 5, Modalities, helps you answer that key question, "What kind of workout should I do and how should I do it?"

Part 6, Feeding Your Body, discusses the importance of nutrition, portion control, hydration, and vitamins. To keep your body running smoothly, you will need the right kind of fuel.

Part 7, Get Going, shows some basic ways to actually start moving your body so that you can put in action everything in this book.

Part 8, The Right Stuff, is primarily about attitude. Like the great Vince Lombardi, you can set yourself up for victory by motivating yourself, striving for excellence, and going after everything you want in life, starting with great fitness and health.

While you could read *Getting Healthy* in any order, we recommend reading it from beginning to end. There is an arc, a logical progression, to the lessons.

The stories in this book are true. They are about real people: people who have the same job you have; people who have been in the same situations as you; people who decided to take the simple steps to change their lives.

The primary objective of this book is to get you moving. That's it. To that end, here are the only three things you really need to do:

1. Read this book.
2. Consult a physician.
3. Start moving your body.

It's time to go get what you want and be the person you want to be. Millions of people have done it before, so we know it's possible. All of the information and technology you need is available.

The only thing stopping you is you.

How badly do you want it?

Part 1

Exercise, Fitness, and Health

Officer Smith Reinvents Himself

Nothing diminishes anxiety faster than action.
~ Walter Anderson

Nobody can go back and start a new beginning,
but anyone can start today and make a new ending.
~ Maria Robinson

John's weight problem started when he was about eight years old. He began eating excessively out of boredom.

This habit continued throughout high school. Despite his weight, he was always very athletic and actually faster than many of his classmates. For a couple of years in college, he slimmed down and was muscular and healthy, but right before graduation, he began eating again.

Even with the additional weight, he was still athletic and passed an obstacle course test to get his first job as a police officer. In the first five years on the job, his weight fluctuated between 230 and 280. Despite being an officer, he was very insecure and always doubted himself and continued to turn to food for comfort.

At 28, he successfully maintained his weight at around 230 for about a year. Shortly after that he met his future wife and began to pack on the pounds. By the time he got married, John was thirty years old and 300 lbs. His insecurity increased when he bought a house and had two kids.

Working at a job he only barely tolerated added to the stress. He had a family to support, and his wife only had a part-time job so she could be home to raise the children.

John always ate a lot when he was in his car or office. He ballooned to 340 lbs. and, before he knew it, 400 was closing in fast.

He had always planned to lose weight but, as with most things in his life, he procrastinated. He would say to himself, "I'll start tomorrow," and then head to a pizza buffet to celebrate his upcoming diet.

He came to realize that he needed to make a change. But he didn't change overnight, and didn't try to; he understood that it would require a shift in lifestyle and not simply a "diet."

His first step was to stop eating in the car on his way home before dinner. He started avoiding foods (like his beloved pizza) that were triggers to eat more, and began to eat fresh fruit and vegetables.

One of the most important steps John took was to dramatically reduce portion size, which included changing his habit of always taking second and third helpings.

Then, he replaced his insecurities with activities, hobbies, and chores, which reduced his fears and decreased his need to rely on food for comfort.

At the time of this writing, John is in his late 40s, has lost 100 lbs., and is on his way to losing another 100. He has gone from two blood pressure medicines to one; he's off all cholesterol medicine and will soon be off his diabetes medication. John no longer experiences heartburn and acid reflux, and he has a lot more energy.

John didn't realize that his weight loss would have a lot of "side effects," like better relationships with his wife and kids; a shift in his attitude and outlook; and the emergence of an ambition he never knew existed before.

Along the way, John experienced his share of setbacks. But, he realized that his failure to stay on target didn't mean that he had to quit outright as he frequently did in the past.

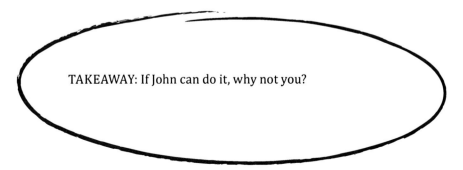

TAKEAWAY: If John can do it, why not you?

The Demands of the Job

The greatest weapon against stress is our ability to choose one thought over another.

~ William James

Law enforcement officers are dedicated public servants who are sworn to protect public safety at any time and place that the peace is threatened.

~ Barbara Boxer

"Long periods of boredom punctuated by moments of sheer terror." That's a common description of police work. Law enforcement is one of the few jobs where an individual can go from 0 to 10 on the action meter in a split second.

You're calmly having a cup of coffee getting ready for your day and in the next moment you're called on to run out the door after a suspect. And it doesn't always work out as successfully as it does in the movies or on television, where officers with 12 lbs. of gear around their waists and 4 lbs. of Kevlar around their torsos are able to chase down a fast-moving suspect that had a pretty decent head start.

You have to ask yourself a very basic question: "Am I ready for this kind of scenario?"

You spend many hours on the shooting range honing your firearm skills, which is important. But the fact of the matter is many officers will go through their entire career and never use their service weapon.

Despite the attention your weapon gets in the movies, your body is actually your most important piece of equipment the vast majority of the time.

Of course, it's not every day that you'll get into a foot chase or a scuffle. But, just as you need to be prepared to respond with deadly force, you also have to be prepared to handle a physical altercation.

More than firearms and physical altercations, it's the daily, near-constant vigilance of police work that requires good physical fitness.

The intensity of the job along with the steady release of adrenaline can rob the body of what it needs to function effectively on a daily basis. The result can be chronic stress and exhaustion, among other things.

Police work is draining, exhausting, stress-inducing, and can have serious negative consequences on your body, mood, attitude, and the quality of your responses to situations around you.

Just like your firearm needs to be clean, loaded, and ready to function, your body needs to be prepared as well. Poor preparation can lead to disastrous results.

At the low end of the spectrum, you risk pulled muscles and stomach upset. At the other end are cardiac arrest and its potentially lethal consequences.

A good way of thinking is "hope for the best, prepare for the worst." Prepare all of your equipment and resources for the *possibility* of something occurring.

In one case, a call came over the radio that several members of the local school track team were suspected of shoplifting at a local store. The police arrived and the suspects began to scatter. Members of the track team versus cops on a foot pursuit. Who would you bet on?

Author Matt asked one of the officers involved in the pursuit, "How did that foot chase work out for you?" He said, "Oh yeah, they definitely had the speed to outrun us. We were lucky we had radios and we could keep calling people with fresh legs and dogs to finally get them."

TAKEAWAY: Your body is one of your most important pieces of equipment. Prepare it the best you can.

Lesson 3

Exercise, Fitness, and Health

To enjoy the glow of good health, you must exercise.

~ Gene Tunney

Health is the thing that makes you feel that now is the best time of the year.

~ Franklin Pierce Adams

For many people, the stated goal of exercising is to "get in shape."

But what exactly does it mean to get in shape?

To a 22-year-old college track athlete, getting in shape might mean being able to run a sub-5-minute mile.

To an 82-year-old woman who suffers from osteoporosis and is recovering from hip replacement surgery, getting in shape might simply mean being able to get up and move around more than she is able to now or maybe doing some stretch exercises.

To the administrative police officer who has spent her whole law-enforcement career on the street and is now stuck behind a desk, getting in shape might mean dropping a few pounds or even avoiding a heart attack.

When it comes down to it, when people say they want to "get in shape," they are really asking, "What are the activities I need to do in order to be in better shape than I am now?"

"Getting in shape" primarily has to do with three things: exercise, fitness, and health.

Exercise is physical activity that is planned, structured, and repetitive for the purpose of conditioning any part of the body.

This can include the heart, lungs, and skeletal muscles. The important part of this definition is that it's planned, structured, and repetitive.

Exercise is an important component needed to achieve your goal of improving your fitness and health.

The key word here is "component," as other components, such as nutrition and daily habits, can work in concert with exercise to improve your fitness and health.

For purposes of this book, fitness means being in adequate *physical* condition to carry out your job. Are you fit enough to perform the tasks your job requires of you?

What about those unforeseen emergencies in which you're the only one around to respond? Are you prepared?

What if you suddenly have to chase someone or wrestle a suspect? Can you handle it?

The question of preparation, or readiness to perform these tasks, is an important aspect of this definition.

Health is the state of being free from illness or injury.

Most people would say they're in good overall health. This can also be a bit deceiving since many can claim to be in good health but may be kidding themselves. Your estimation of your health as "good" is often your rationalization for not exercising.

Of course, the state of your health can change quickly. Most of us know what it's like to feel good one day and come down with a major cold or flu the next.

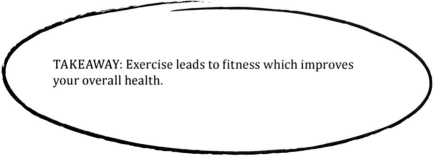

TAKEAWAY: Exercise leads to fitness which improves your overall health.

Exercise and Activity

*It is exercise alone that supports the spirits, and
keeps the mind in vigor.*

~ Marcus Tullius Cicero

*Lack of activity destroys the good condition of every
human being, while movement and methodical
physical exercise save it and preserve it.*

~ Plato

It's important to make a distinction early in the book between exercise and activity.

As we noted in the previous lesson, exercise is purposeful movement with the intent of improving or increasing physical fitness levels and reducing risk of disease. By its very nature, exercise is repetitive, structured, and planned.

Activity is the state or quality of being active or being engaged in lively action or movement.

Yes, being active and moving will burn off calories and help fitness and health levels.

But, exercise is the best way to burn calories and get in shape.

If you follow the guidelines of a proper exercise regimen, you should be exercising for around 30 minutes a day, 3-4 days a week, for a total of about 1.5 hours each week. In this way, you can decrease your risk of several diseases and look and feel better.

However, if you spend 1.5 hours a week exercising, that still leaves 166.5 hours. What you do with that time will impact your fitness and health levels as well. That's where you can increase your activity.

When Matt did some fitness consulting with an energy company, he found that the employees who drove the trucks and climbed the poles had a reasonable level of overall fitness and fairly low body fat.

When they received promotions and were moved to administration and management or into support roles, their fitness levels decreased and their body fat levels increased.

What happened? They went from a somewhat active lifestyle to a sedentary one, and all those calories they burned by being outside performing their job tasks were no longer being burned.

Both exercise and activity are important for maintaining overall physical health.

What is the implication for law enforcement?

Officers on the street are relatively active compared to those who work indoors, of course.

Think of the implications for bike patrol officers. Riding 20-40 miles a day, these individuals burn calories while at work.

Contrast these officers with those who have been promoted to a job where their responsibility for others grows, but their activity level decreases.

Think also of administrative support staff, emergency dispatchers, and others. Sitting at a desk for the majority of the day, these people fall into the "inactive" category.

While a comprehensive exercise program is more important for the inactive group than the active patrol officers generally speaking, all personnel must find a way to increase their activity throughout the day. Exercise on its own is not enough; neither is activity.

TAKEAWAY: A combination of exercise and activity is the best approach for maintaining fitness and health.

The Benefits of Exercise

He who has health, has hope; and he who has hope,
has everything.

~ Thomas Carlyle

Physical fitness is not only one of the most important
keys to a healthy body; it is the basis of
dynamic and creative intellectual activity.

~ John F. Kennedy

Why should you participate in an exercise program? Why can't you just watch what you eat, stay active, and make good decisions? Won't this be enough?

Research has shown that planned, purposeful movement has many benefits over and above simple activity for individuals who engage in it on a regular basis.

Exercise has been shown to reduce the risk of heart disease and several forms of cancer. Proper exercise can decrease the risk of diabetes and hypertension, reduce body fat, and improve your sleep.

An aerobic exercise program will improve your lungs, helping you breathe more easily and become less fatigued during the day.

Resistance exercise makes your bones and muscles stronger so that you can physically perform your job better, as well as decrease your risk for osteoporosis.

Some of the most important benefits of exercise to police officers are rarely discussed, however. Typically, authors focus on the benefits of being stronger and faster and being able to stop a perpetrator.

One of these important benefits is positive effects on the brain.

Exercise can be a cathartic or cleansing experience, allowing you the opportunity to free your mind from daily struggles and stress.

One of Matt's personal training clients once said, "I disagree when you say exercise helps me with my problems. After I work out, the problems are still there!"

That perspective misses the point. Even a single exercise session can shift your attitude, your creativity, your imagination, and your openness so that you are able to see solutions you may not have been able to see before. Of course your problems are still there, but now you're better equipped to solve them.

Want a new perspective on a problem? Go out for a walk or run!

Police officers experience stress in many forms on a daily basis. A proper exercise program can go a long way to reduce stress.

Exercise helps activate endorphins, those "feel good" neurotransmitters released from the brain during exercise. When you exercise, it helps your mind just as much as it helps your body.

In law enforcement, the ability to use one's brain long before physical force — to be clever, to maintain composure, to engage in verbal judo and de-escalate a delicate situation — is of critical importance. And the ability to effectively address stress can be a life saver.

Unfortunately, all too often, officers turn to alcohol, television, an explosive temper, or other unproductive methods of trying to handle their stress.

In reality, these "solutions" serve to exacerbate an officer's stress over the long term.

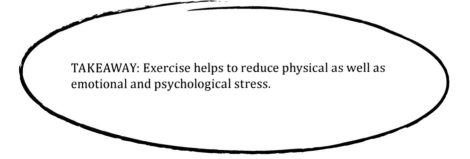

TAKEAWAY: Exercise helps to reduce physical as well as emotional and psychological stress.

Does Exercise Have a Downside?

You have to fight to reach your dream. You have to sacrifice and work hard for it.

~ Lionel Messi

You aren't going to find anybody that's going to be successful without making a sacrifice and without perseverance.

~ Lou Holtz

As beneficial as exercise is, it's important to be aware that there are times exercise may not be the best medicine under certain conditions.

Exercise can be a potent stimulus for developing myocardial ischemia. This means that during exercise, blood flow to the heart can actually decrease, indicating a potential problem.

During a stress test, the doctor has you exercise during the EKG because the heart reacts differently when it's exercising as opposed to when it's not. Potential problems will manifest themselves while the body is under stress.

During Matt's tenure as a fitness club owner, several serious cardiovascular incidents occurred. All of these incidents happened before Automatic External Defibrillators (AED) were readily available.

One incident involved a member who "fell out" one morning while exercising. The club staff and members performed CPR and were able to stabilize him until the ambulance arrived. He recovered and lived another 25 years with the help of an implanted Automatic Internal Defibrillator (AID).

In another incident, a man Matt was working out collapsed. Matt performed CPR until emergency services arrived. Unfortunately, the man did not survive, but the man's wife thanked Matt for all he did since she knew he lived longer than he would have had he not been exercising.

Be sure to consult your doctor before beginning any exercise program.

Astronaut Neil Armstrong was quoted as saying, "I believe that every human has a finite amount of heartbeats. I don't intend to waste any of mine running around doing exercises." The first man on the moon may have been a bit off on this one.

Even if you do have a finite number of beats, the long-term effect of exercise will actually make your heart more efficient, lowering your Resting Heart Rate (RHR). Therefore, while you may increase your heart rate during exercise, you are "paying it forward" with a lower rate the rest of your time.

Athletes have an RHR of around 44 beats per minute. The average RHR in an untrained individual is 72 beats per minute. Do the math over an average lifetime. Bit of a savings over time, isn't there?

An aspect of exercise that may be deemed a downside is that it takes time, plain and simple. Matt knows of several relationships (including an early one of his own) that dissolved because an individual was spending too much time at the gym.

In addition, a lot of accidents happen in the gym. The weight room is, by its nature, a dangerous place. Steel objects flying about with a great deal of force; inattentiveness and crowded conditions can potentially lead to serious situations. Gym rules are meant to be followed, but just like everyone in law enforcement knows, not all rules are followed all the time.

With exercise there is always potential for negative consequences. And like any other decision you make, the decision to exercise will include sacrifice, saying no to one thing in order to say yes to something else.

TAKEAWAY: Be aware of your own situation and the potential risks of exercise.

Part 2

Facing Fear

Are You Afraid of Exercise?

By changing nothing, nothing changes.

~ Tony Robbins

*A year from now you will wish
you had started today.*

~ Karen Lamb

Are you afraid of exercise, fitness, and health?

This may seem like a strange question, but so many people spend so much time avoiding getting healthy that you might have to ask if there's any fear involved.

By the way, here's a funny thing about fear: Often people who are afraid don't even realize that fear is the thing standing in their way. It often masks itself as something else, like procrastination.

What is your fear? Not knowing where to start? Not knowing what to do or how long to do it? Thinking it will be too hard? Feeling you can't make time to exercise without taking something away from someone or something else? How about the fear of spending a lot of time exercising and not getting results?

Your fear may have you so locked down that you just can't get away from the television. Maybe you've convinced yourself that after a long shift you're just too tired to exercise. Or that you're too busy. (Check out Dr. Joe Serio's book, *Time Management: 50 Lessons on Finding Time for What's Important.*)

You may think you don't have the discipline to stay committed to an exercise program once you get started. Or that you're too far gone to exercise at this stage in your life: You're too old, too overweight, or your sweet tooth is just too powerful.

As law enforcement officers, you may be most afraid of getting sick, injured, or dying. You may be afraid that something will happen to you, and your children may not be properly cared for financially, or your spouse will have to go on without you.

Many times, it's the fear of other, more deeply-rooted things that keep you from exercising:

- Feelings that nothing you ever do turns out right.
- Feelings that you can never have what other people have.
- Feelings from childhood that you can't be successful and so you undermine your own efforts.

Many of these fears, you would think, would drive you to get in shape and exercise regularly. And that's exactly what some people do.

For most people, though, this isn't the case. Even when the consequences of inaction can be serious, you stick to what you know — whether it's good for you or not. A body at rest tends to stay at rest and all that.

You're a creature of habit, and facing fears means changing habits.

It's time to identify clearly why it is you're resisting exercise and getting fit. It's time to examine your justifications and rationalizations to see what stands behind them.

In the next lesson, we're going to look at the core of your fear and how it might be impacting your exercise, fitness, and health.

TAKEAWAY: Fear may be keeping you from having the fitness and health you want and deserve.

The Fear List

The greatest mistake a man can make is to be afraid of making one.

~ Elbert Hubbard

Failure is an inescapable part of life and a critically important part of any successful life.

~ Tal Ben-Shahar

Let's dive a little bit deeper into this issue of fear.

What is it?

In a broad sense, fear is an unpleasant emotion caused by the belief that someone or something is dangerous, likely to cause pain, is a threat, or is unpleasant.

Ask people what they are afraid of and frequently the first things you'll hear includes spiders, snakes, heights, and the dentist.

Probe a little deeper and the list of fears becomes more delicate, more sensitive, and a little more profound. Facial expressions change to reveal more intimate secrets. People appear more childlike, as if they are being transported to an earlier moment in time when those fears were initially experienced. At the same time, they look weary from hanging on to those fears for a very long time.

The list becomes predictable and very familiar:

- Fear of making mistakes
- Fear of rejection

- Fear of embarrassment
- Fear of criticism
- Fear of losing approval/love
- Fear of losing control
- Fear of failure
- Fear of success

The problem, of course, isn't the presence of fear. The problem is how you handle fear, what you do with it. There are plenty of successful men and women who feel fear but are not fearful. They are not paralyzed by fear.

In the list above, the focus of power and energy in most of those fears lies with someone else. You give away your power, worrying what others will think of you, letting them judge you and determine your path, instead of living life on your own terms.

Now think about the list of fears in terms of exercise, fitness, and health:

- How have the fears listed above influenced what you eat, how you eat, how much you eat, and when you eat?
- How much time have you wasted wringing your hands over the thought of exercising?
- How many times have you started exercising half-heartedly only to stop within weeks, maybe even days?
- How many times have you stopped yourself from going to the gym because you're self-conscious about how you'd look compared to other people?
- How has fear been driving your decisions?

Start pondering the role fear might be playing in your attitude toward exercise, fitness, and health.

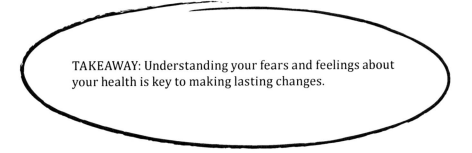

TAKEAWAY: Understanding your fears and feelings about your health is key to making lasting changes.

Lesson 9

Putting Off Exercise

When we can no longer change a situation, we are challenged to change ourselves.

~ Viktor Frankl

I don't run away from a challenge because I am afraid. Instead, I run toward it because the only way to escape fear is to trample it beneath your feet.

~ Nadia Comaneci

When you're afraid of exercise, you'll find a way to justify why you don't do it. In fact, for as long as there's been exercise, people have found excuses not to do it. Often, those excuses feel like reasons, but they're not.

We can break the excuses down into three general categories:

1. A simple choice not to do it. You've made a decision that for whatever reason — lazy, don't feel like it, set in your ways — you will not exercise. We can provide all of the research showing the vast benefits of simple exercise, but we can't make you do it. You can lead a horse to water....

2. The dreaded "Toos." Why don't you work out? You're too busy. You're too tired. You're legs are too achy, your back is too sore. The equipment at the department is too lousy. It's too cold. It's too hot. You're too old. It's too expensive.

3. An attempt to substitute something else in exercise's place. "I play golf so I don't need to exercise." "I work in the garden so that serves as my workout." "I walk enough on my shift." As we've already mentioned, there's a significant difference between activity and exercise.

If you're making excuses like the ones above, take a moment to realize the cost of continuing to treat these excuses like they are valid reasons:

- You say you don't have time to exercise, but surely you will find time to be sick.
- You say it's too expensive, but the cost of staying at a hospital is sky high.
- You say the gym is too far away, but you can start by simply walking around the block.

The first step in exercising is to get real with yourself. Matt recently started a 91-year-old man on an exercise program. He was doing leg presses with 90 lbs., so Matt added one pound to the resistance so the client would be lifting his age!

What's your excuse again?

The second step is to evaluate the environment you work in. Part of your lifestyle is influenced by your position in the department and your level of activity and exercise.

Officers on the street, perhaps especially those on bike patrol or SWAT, will get much more activity and exercise than administrative officers or dispatchers sitting behind a desk or console all day.

The third step is to realize that exercise will provide the fitness and health you need and greatly reduce reliance on medication to fix what ails you.

Many, if not most, illnesses and disease can be reversed or slowed by sufficient exercise, adequate nutrition, and an overall healthy lifestyle. Most people need to be active more than they need their doctors. Remember Officer Smith in Lesson 1? He's living proof.

The excuses for not staying in shape are endless. It's up to you to start facing your excuses and decide what's really important to you. When you get clear about that, incorporating an exercise program into your life will become much easier.

TAKEAWAY: Your excuses for not exercising are keeping you from getting what you need and want.

Handling Your Fear

We fear something before we hate it; a child who fears noises becomes a man who hates noises.

~ Cyril Connolly

How we relate to fear determines how we do in life, and maybe it is the essence of who we are.

~ Thom Rutledge

What is your fear saying to you? If you look at the list of fears in Lesson 8, you could summarize it as "I can't handle it."

- I can't handle the possibility of being embarrassed.
- I can't handle the possibility of being criticized.
- I can't handle the possibility of being rejected.
- I can't handle the possibility of failing.

Many people's response to this mantra of "I can't handle it" frequently is to give mediocre performances instead of doing their best or simply not try at all. They're too busy protecting themselves. They're so afraid of the possibility of feeling fear and pain that they treat it as though it's guaranteed.

You can spend years "protecting yourself" from the possibility of criticism and failure. You focus on your shortcomings, your imperfections, and the opinions of others. You convince yourself you can't handle most things. But, that which you focus on expands and becomes reality.

The sad part is your imagination is bubbling with wonderful things you want to do and be, even if it's simply to get in better shape, be healthier, and have more time with your family.

It doesn't require a sudden, dramatic event in your life to make you believe you can't handle it. It's already happened, slowly, subtly. You created the responses a long time ago every time you thought you couldn't handle something, every time you thought you weren't good enough.

You play your responses over and over again in your head. "I'll never get in shape." "I can never lose weight." "I don't deserve to look good." "I've never really been successful at anything."

The protective layers built up over the years have pushed in the walls of your comfort zone closer and closer to the point you don't want to risk very much or take too many chances, if any. In many cases, those walls have also become so thick that breaking through them can be difficult.

Facing fear means starting to understand you can handle much more than you believe you can.

Facing fear means crafting for yourself a new story about your past, one that changes your beliefs, your assumptions, your thoughts, and your responses.

You can deal with the fear of exercising, getting fit, and being healthy not by dancing around it or eliminating it, but by going through it — having courage to act not in the absence of fear but in spite of it.

Contrary to what you might be feeling, you don't have to do it alone, you don't have to reinvent the wheel, and you don't have to suffer in silence. Lack of knowledge and experience is not weakness, it's a starting point.

You will not be the first person to face your issues around exercise, fitness, and health. Many others have done it before, and you can, too. You can handle it.

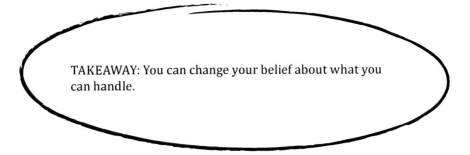

TAKEAWAY: You can change your belief about what you can handle.

Why Law Enforcement Joined Matt's Club

Success depends upon previous preparation, and without such preparation there is sure to be failure.

~ Confucius

The proactive approach to a mistake is to acknowledge it instantly, correct and learn from it.

~ Stephen Covey

In the late 1970s, Matt was finishing up his undergraduate degree in law enforcement at a university in Texas, but he didn't really see his future going in that direction.

He joined a fitness club that had revolutionary exercise equipment known as Nautilus machines. He was immediately astounded by the effectiveness of the equipment and sensed his career path changing to an exercise and fitness emphasis.

He spent so much time at the club they offered him a job. Shortly after, through a series of "right place right time" adventures, he bought that club.

At the tender age of 21, Matt became a business owner. Armed with his degree in law enforcement and very little business knowledge, he ventured into the health club world.

He used a lot of different kinds of marketing to get the club's name out to the public. Radio ads reached some ears and newspaper ads reached some eyes.

The best advertising, of course, was word of mouth. If a member was happy, they'd bring their friends to the club.

And word of mouth was the best source of advertising in almost every population except one: the law enforcement community.

Yes, police officers would bring their friends in to work out, but they didn't join at the same time or for the same reasons as other people.

They didn't get a membership in January as part of their New Year's resolution, only to fall dormant a month or two later. And they didn't get memberships when they were still fresh, eager young cops out of the academy.

Police officers would generally join the club when their fear was greatest: *after* they had been in a fight with a suspect and were embarrassed by the results. Or maybe they had been in a foot pursuit and couldn't keep up, winded, achy, and defeated.

Getting embarrassed out on the streets and being unable to perform at a sufficient level was apparently the factor convincing them they needed some additional fitness training in order to perform their jobs. See the fear at work here?

Seeing this happen time and time again, even at his young age, Matt kept thinking that perhaps proactivity is a better approach than reactivity. Officers need some level of fitness to deal not only with day-to-day situations, but also life-and-death situations.

An officer's fitness level affects his or her own well-being and that of his or her partner. If you're an active police officer, at some point you may be in a tactical situation that requires some level of fitness: strength, cardiovascular endurance, or flexibility.

Don't let fear of any kind stop you from getting in the shape you need to be in on the streets.

TAKEAWAY: Don't wait for disaster to strike before preparing for it.

Part 3

Creating a System

Lesson 12
Belief: The Key to Your Success

All that we are is the result of what we have thought.

~ Buddha

It's not who you are that holds you back, it's who you think you're not.

~ Unknown

Most people skip the most important part of getting what they want: believing that it's possible. Belief is one of the cornerstones of achieving goals.

Did you used to make New Year's resolutions? If so, perhaps you stuck with them for a few days, weeks, or even months. But a year was just too long. You ran out of enthusiasm. You got bored. You ultimately told yourself the goal didn't matter that much, so it was no big deal if you stopped chasing it.

And yet, year after year, you made the resolutions. And, year after year, you got the same results. You didn't do a fraction of the things you told yourself you would do. The way you lived your life didn't support reaching the goals because you didn't truly think they were possible.

Lacking the belief that something is possible actually means it is not possible. To paraphrase Henry Ford, if you think you can, you're right. If you think you can't, you're right.

The belief "I can" helps you clearly define the goal and create a system for getting it. And having a clearly defined goal and system reinforces your belief in the project, especially when the going gets difficult.

You can go through the motions as much as you want. You can talk about exercising, getting fit, and being healthy. You can buy countless books about how to do it. But if you don't believe it, if you don't believe in it, if you don't believe in yourself, how do you expect to actually get it?

A critical part of exercise, fitness, and health that most people don't think about is that sometimes it requires you to dive deep into yourself, especially if you've been putting it off for years.

Think about the fitness goals you set for yourself that you didn't reach. Now think about the underlying beliefs you had around those goals. It might have looked something like this:

Goal: I'm going to lose weight.

Belief: I can't lose weight. I've never succeeded at anything.

Belief: I've tried before and it never worked.

Belief: I don't deserve to be healthy and happy because people always told me I'm no good.

According to scores of successful people — that is, people who reach their goals and live their dreams — the number one most important ingredient in reaching success is perseverance. But it's difficult to face the tough times and work through them if you don't believe in what you're doing or its possibility for success.

How many times have you given up on something when it got difficult?

How many times have you given up on something because your heart wasn't in it?

How many times have you given up on something because you just didn't believe you could have it?

Decide what you believe, without judgment or conclusions, without worrying about the road ahead, without worrying about what other people will say, or worrying about failing.

Pick an exercise, fitness, and health goal you can believe in. Make it small at first, if necessary. The rest of the book will show you how to get it.

TAKEAWAY: Your belief in yourself and the task before you is critical to your success.

Lesson 13

Determine Your Priorities

Action expresses priorities.

~ Mahatma Gandhi

Desires dictate our priorities, priorities shape our choices, and choices determine our actions.

~ Dallin H. Oaks

What's important to you?

When you determine what's truly important, it becomes possible to decide what you're going to sacrifice in order to get it.

If you don't know, you may sacrifice the wrong thing.

For example, if you declare that exercise, fitness, and health are important to you but you spend your exercise time watching television, you have sacrificed the wrong thing.

If you don't proactively determine your priorities, you will actually still have priorities but they may not lead you to a place you want to go.

For example, if you say you're going to exercise and lose weight, but instead you spend hours in front of the television and you eat three pizzas a week, watching television and eating pizza are, in reality, your priorities.

So often you declare your priorities and yet your actions don't reflect your words. And, by the way, there's no need to declare your priorities to the world; you will show the world your priorities by what you do.

As with belief, establishing your priorities is not an exercise in a vacuum to be done for its own sake. It is a necessary part of moving forward to get what you want. It's the foundation for achieving goals.

In the early 1980s, Matt completed the Ironman Triathlon (2.4 mile swim, 112 mile bike ride, and a 26.2 mile run). If you looked at Matt and the other competitors, you could easily determine what their priorities had been for at least the previous 4-6 months. If competing in the Ironman competition wasn't a priority, they wouldn't have stuck to it when the training got tough.

After the race, Matt was approached by a newspaper reporter who very casually said, "The Ironman? I was thinking about doing that once." That hit a nerve. Matt wanted to tell the guy, "You have no idea how much I have sweated, suffered, bled, lost relationships, and lost time to train for this race. This race defined me in my 20s. You've got to do more than just think about it."

There are a couple of reasons you have to make exercise, fitness, and health a priority if you want to enjoy the benefits they bring:

- First, it's not simple. If it were, everyone would do it.
- Second, there are always competing activities, interruptions, and distractions that threaten to take time away from your priorities. You have to protect the time you create to pursue your priorities. If it's not a priority, you won't do it.

Successful people get what they want because they're very good at understanding those two things.

Author Joe always had a difficult time losing weight. He finally made it a priority and carved out the time to exercise and change his eating habits. He lost 17 lbs. in six weeks with little stress, difficulty, or anxiety.

Once it became a priority, losing the weight was a relatively easy goal to reach.

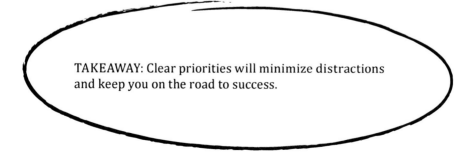

TAKEAWAY: Clear priorities will minimize distractions and keep you on the road to success.

Lesson 14

Visualization: See Your Future

*Dare to visualize a world in which your most
treasured dreams have become true.*

~ Ralph Marston

*If you want to reach a goal, you must 'see the
reaching' in your own mind
before you actually arrive at your goal.*

~ Zig Ziglar

Once you believe in and prioritize something, it becomes much easier to plan for it and move forward. The next step after belief and prioritizing is visualization.

It took Joe a long time to trust this process. When people said he should visualize where he wanted to go — "If you can see it, you can be it" — it sounded like New Age, warm and fuzzy, hocus pocus.

He came to understand that visualizing isn't simply about picturing an object or an outcome; it's picturing yourself actually doing something. It's about experiencing the feeling of accomplishing that thing *before you do it*. Your brain doesn't know the difference between the imagined accomplishment and the real one. When you step up to do it in "real life," you have already practiced it and accomplished it in your mind.

The golf great Jack Nicklaus said that before he ever took a swing, whether in practice or in competition, he always visualized the ball "sitting high and pretty and white up on the green."

Arnold Schwarzenegger said of becoming Mr. Universe, "I pictured myself on that top spot on the podium, winning first place."

A few years ago, Joe thought it would be great to play in a band on the world famous 6th Street in Austin, known as the Live Music Capital of the World. But his brain couldn't visualize it for two simple reasons:

- First, he didn't believe he could do it. The old voice in his head kicked in, saying, "You can't play with them. You're not good enough." He had little belief.

- Second, he had never been to 6th Street, or even to Austin for that matter.

The first step in helping him visualize his own performance on 6th Street was to go there and see the bands that were playing. Having a picture in his mind of what 6th Street looked like, he could easily visualize himself playing there. This cemented the belief, and he knew right then he would do it someday.

A year and a half later, he moved to Austin, and a month after that he had his first experience playing on 6th Street.

This process works for exercise, fitness, and health as well. When you have belief, priority, and vision connected to your goals, you improve the likelihood that your goals — and your dreams — will come true.

Most people don't take the time to visualize, and, not coincidentally, most people never get what they really want or need.

Belief and visualization spring directly from three key questions you should ask yourself: **Who am I? What do I want? How am I going to get it?** The more specific the answers, the easier it is to visualize.

Take the time to visualize how you want to look and how, in fact, you *will* look. Visualize being more active, more mobile, and having more energy. Visualize your improved family life after you get fit — think about the activities you'll be able to do with your loved ones. Soon, you'll find you start to think better, and then you'll start to act better, making new choices that line up with your goals.

TAKEAWAY: We create twice, first in our minds and then in reality. See your future and then go get it.

Decide, Commit, Succeed

Do or do not. There is no try.

~ Yoda

Until one is committed, there is hesitancy,
the chance to draw back. Whatever you can do or
dream you can, begin it. Boldness has genius, power,
and magic in it. Begin it now.

~ Johann Wolfgang von Goethe

You may have already dreamed about things you want, expressed a desire to live a better life, to get in great shape, to eat well, and feel fantastic. You may have made some good choices in the past.

You may have even clarified exactly what you want and how you were going to get it.

And then you might've changed your mind. Maybe you got bored with what you were doing and distracted by the new shiny object that came into sight.

You set yourself up for failure by skipping the process of deciding and committing.

Joe used to be a procrastinator. When he was heavily weighed down by it, he would watch countless hours of television. He even watched infomercials for things like P90X, the extreme exercise workout regimen.

Fortunately, something good came out of it. He was inspired by the tagline of Beach Body, the parent company of P90X: *Decide. Commit. Succeed.*®

This tagline is a simple reminder you can memorize and carry with you at all times to keep yourself on track. Here's how to use it.

Ask yourself: "Have I truly decided what I want?"

Don't take this word "decided" too lightly. You either decide or you don't decide; there is no in-between. Unfortunately, you may "decide" several times a week and end up doing nothing: "I'm going to exercise. I changed my mind, I'm not going to exercise. I'm going to jog. No, I'm going to lift weights. I'm going to work out every day. Ok, maybe only once a month." That's not deciding.

Either you've decided or you haven't. You can't have it both ways.

While deciding is critically important, it's not enough.

Once you've decided you want to be in charge of your life, that you are ready to deal with your fear, get in shape, and be healthy, you then ask yourself: "Am I committed to it?"

Think about this: Five frogs are sitting on a log. One decides to jump off. How many frogs are left? The answer, of course, is five. The frog that decided to jump did just that: decided. He didn't actually jump. You can decide all you want, but, until you act, your decisions don't mean very much.

You can't be committed to an undertaking and not committed at the same time.

You can't be committed to exercise and only do it once or twice a month. You can't be committed to health and continue to smoke or eat lots of junk food.

A commitment is not simply a promise that you're going to do something. It is the action itself. You display your commitment in the regular, consistent doing of a thing.

When you decide and commit, the succeed part will take care of itself. Before you know it, you will be reaching your goals and creating the kind of life you really want.

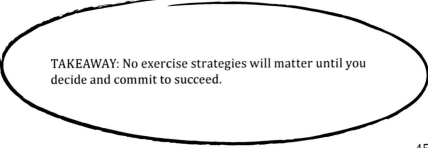

TAKEAWAY: No exercise strategies will matter until you decide and commit to succeed.

How to Set Goals

*Setting goals is the first step in turning the
invisible into the visible.*

~ Tony Robbins

*What you get by achieving your goals
is not as important as what you become by
achieving your goals.*

~ Johann Wolfgang von Goethe

Once you have clarified your beliefs and determined your priorities, it will be easier to identify exactly where you want to go. If you have determined that fitness and health are truly something you value, you then need to decide what that looks like and how you're going to get it.

After all, if you don't know where you're headed, you'll end up going wherever life takes you.

You need a goal and a plan to reach that goal.

Whether you realize it or not, that plan started to take shape when you asked yourself the three core questions: **Who am I? What do I want? How am I going to get it?**

Ultimately, when you do make your goals, it's critical to understand the difference between real goals and fake goals.

Fake goals are vague hopes, desires, and wishes — things that are very difficult to attain because there's nothing concrete about them. They're typically empty statements with no context or substance: "I want to lose weight."

"I want to get in shape." "I want to be healthy." Fake goals are resistant to planning.

Setting real goals forces you to get very practical, specific, and action-oriented. It requires you to get very real.

SMART is a simple acronym you can use to create real rather than fake goals. SMART goals are the difference between wishful thinking and making real progress.

S — Specific. Your goal has to be as specific as possible. "I want to lose weight" is not a real goal. "I am going to lose 15 lbs. between January 1st and February 15th, and here's how I'm going to do it" is a much more powerful goal, making it more difficult for you to be thrown off course.

M — Measurable. You have to know exactly what it is, exactly what you are trying to do. How will you know when you've reached the goal? What does "done" look like? In our weight-loss example, done is when the person loses 15 lbs.

A — Attainable. Is it actually possible to reach this goal? Losing 100 lbs. in a week is not attainable, but losing 15 in 6 weeks is within reach. (Understand the realities of your situation and set your goals in consultation with your doctor. Don't hurt yourself by trying to do too much too fast.)

R — Results-oriented. You need to set goals like you set a destination when you get in the car — with the expectation you will get there. The pursuit of goals is critical, but you can easily forget that you actually need to arrive at your destination.

T — Time-bound. In the weight-loss example above, the time limit was six weeks. Deadlines are critical when pursuing goals.

When you set SMART goals, you create the context for the goals. You provide them with the framework that makes them easier to attain.

TAKEAWAY: Be SMART. Don't fool yourself into thinking that you have real goals if you don't.

Lesson 17
Make SMART Goals SMARTER

Arise! Awake! And stop not until the goal is reached.

~ Swami Vivekananda

*Courage — the quality of daring to crawl out from
under the covers to respond to fear with
fresh attention and appropriate responses.*

~ Sarah Quigley

The simplest way to make a SMART goal more effective is to make it SMARTER. Here's how.

E — Evaluate. After you've set your goal, build in an evaluation phase.

The primary function of the evaluation stage, of course, is to see if everything is going according to plan, if everything has been done correctly, if you're still on target for an on-time completion, and if anything needs to be fixed or improved. For example, you may have started out too ambitious and hurt yourself, requiring some down time and re-evaluation of your workout.

Depending on the goal and the plan, evaluation could be weekly, monthly, or quarterly. When talking about exercise, fitness, and health, evaluation can come at the end of every day. Did you eat well that day? Did you take a walk, jog, or lift weights that day? Did you take the day off from exercise? Did you stick to your plan and pursue your goals?

A timely evaluation will tell you if you need to change tactics within the pursuit of your goal in order to stay on track.

Your evaluation also may show that your original goal was too ambitious and simply couldn't be reached in a certain time frame or under certain conditions. Frequently, you set goals that require more time than you first anticipated.

R — Re-do. Sometimes this can be the hardest part. After you've gone down the road toward the goal and have done the evaluation, you realize parts of your approach need to be changed, adjusted, or re-done. It can be difficult to find the energy and patience, especially if it has been a hard slog to get to your current point.

This is probably a good time in the process to take a break, if you have that luxury. It could be a few hours or a day or two to recharge your batteries and get into the right frame of mind. In many cases, it will require devising a plan to handle the adjustment portion of your goal.

For example, when Officer Smith, portrayed in Lesson 1, was in the process of losing weight, his evaluation told him he needed to re-do his goal statement.

His progress wasn't as fast as he anticipated. In the past, he would have simply quit trying, but now that he had a plan in place, he reconsidered his approach and made the necessary changes.

The bottom line is this: What will you do if you fall off the wagon? What's your plan for getting back to exercising and improving your health after the holidays or after you've been sick?

It helps to build a cushion of time into your original plan so that when the re-do phase arrives — and it does quite often — you have the flexibility to adjust and adapt without letting frustration take over.

Developing SMARTER goals helps reduce fear, keep you on track, and get you to your goal faster than you would otherwise.

TAKEAWAY: Don't worry if things don't go exactly as planned. Re-evaluate, stay flexible, and make changes.

Set Yourself Up for Success

The starting point of all success is desire.

~ Napoleon Hill

*Success consists of going from failure to failure
without loss of enthusiasm.*

~ Winston Churchill

All of the information you need to know to lose weight, get fit, and be healthy is readily available, whether through a doctor, nutritionist, fitness trainer, books, or the internet.

You can easily find out what exercises to do and what foods to eat. Don't get bogged down with how many different opinions there are out there — choose what works best for you and stick with it.

As with most activities, the challenge lies not in the knowing but in the doing.

Exercising, getting fit, and staying healthy is often a psychological game.

Are you motivated to do it? Will you have the determination to do it when you're tired and just want to go back to bed? Will you pass up that pizza or dessert when you've committed to losing weight? What kinds of excuses will you rely on to rationalize not doing what you should?

Successful people set themselves up for success. They create conditions that minimize the possibility of failure while taking steps to maximize the probability of success.

Here are some suggestions that may help you deal with the psychological challenge of going after your exercise, fitness, and health goals:

- For many people, eating unhealthy food is a central part of their health issues. Go through your pantry and refrigerator and clear out the junk food, ice cream, and other things that keep you stuck in your bad habits.

  You can't eat it if it's not there.

- Tell someone about your goals and ask them to help you stay on track. Any task is easier when you have an accountability partner.

  Better yet, if you have someone to go through the process with you, it becomes that much easier to muster the psychological strength to keep going when you want to stop.

- Make sure you have what you need to get started. Whether its clothing, footwear, a bicycle, weights, or even a gym membership, make sure you have the right tools to make your task easier and that everything is in working order.

  Being prepared helps reduce the fear of pursuing your goal.

- It will be easier to be committed to a program if you assign a specific time to do it and make it a part of your day. Use your calendar to schedule your workout sessions. If it's possible to work out at the same time every day, it will be easier to develop it into a habit.

  Before long, you'll find yourself wanting to work out.

- Don't use being tired as an excuse. You may feel physically tired when you're sitting still, but the act of getting your body moving, even after a long day, will give you enough energy to get through the workout. You'll feel better about having stepped up to the challenge.

  Even if you're too exhausted to do your regular routine, it's better to have done something than nothing.

TAKEAWAY: Set yourself up for success by getting rid of temptations and enlisting support from your friends or family.

Creating a System

A bad system will beat a good person every time.

~ W. Edwards Deming

Systems are not sexy — but they really do drive everything we do!

~ Carrie Wilkerson

The mechanisms you put in place to make it easier to be healthy will make up your system — and your system is critical to your success.

When you walk into a Subway sandwich shop, you see a system at work. The employees say the same thing every time — "Welcome to Subway!" — and they always ask you the same questions: "What kind of bread do you want? Do you want cheese? Do you want it toasted?"

They have a process supported by containers so they don't have to search for anything while they're building a sandwich. Everything is laid out in a predictable fashion to increase efficiency and help them serve more customers.

When the employees are juggling multiple customers, they use the containers and processes that make up their system to help manage their tasks so they don't have to think too much. They just do it.

They are successful because they set up a system.

You can do the same thing in your life. When you use containers and processes to create a system, you make it easier to reach your goals.

Make sure everything you need is in its proper place, in its proper container.

You don't want to have to look for your car keys when you're headed out to the gym. Put them in the same place every time.

You don't want to have to look for the bicycle pump if your tires need inflating.

Same with your clothes, weights, and anything else you need to work out. Don't defeat your efforts by being disorganized.

Put your workout times on your calendar. If you don't make exercise a priority, you won't do it. It can't be an afterthought; it has to be built into your life.

Be aware of portion size. When you have a typical dinner plate, the temptation is to fill it up. Use a smaller plate when eating dinner and eat more slowly. You may be tempted to say that you'll simply fill up the smaller plate two or three times, but when you combine smaller portions with a slower eating pace, you allow your body time to feel full.

When you go out to dinner, request a to-go box when you order your meal and immediately put half of it in there. Restaurant portion sizes are much larger than a recommended serving size.

Also, you can automatically say no when the waiter asks if you want dessert. Don't take time to think about it. This is especially useful if you have a huge sweet tooth and dessert is your downfall.

Decide you're going to take the stairs whenever possible. If you work on the second or third floor of your building, walk. It may not feel significant, but it will keep your body moving and that is one of the keys to overall good health.

When you decide and commit to all of this in advance, you don't have to think very much when it comes to working out and saying no to things that keep you from reaching your goal. These mechanisms will become habit before long and require less and less willpower.

TAKEAWAY: Put a system in place that streamlines your process to reach your goals.

Lesson 20

Great Questions to Help You Reach Your Goal

You are never too old to set another goal or to dream a new dream.

~ C. S. Lewis

The difference between who you are and who you want to be is what you do.

~ Bill Phillips

Write down one exercise, fitness, or health goal you are going to achieve.

You can assess the quality of your goal with a series of questions.

Why do I want to pursue this goal?

Is it something I really want to do for myself or am I doing it because others expect it of me? Am I doing it because it will bring me fame and fortune and people will think highly of me? Am I doing it because it's of great importance to me and it doesn't matter what other people think?

Am I pursuing this particular goal because I have nothing better to do? Because I don't know what else to do? Because I really don't know what I'm interested in?

Does pursuing this goal get me closer to the overall lifestyle I want to have for myself? Does this goal feed into my overall plan? Do I even have an overall plan? Does pursuing this goal take away from more important goals or priorities I have in life?

54

What direct benefits do I expect to get out of pursuing and reaching this goal? What things may become possible when I reach this goal?

Is the goal Specific? Measurable? Attainable? Results-oriented? Time-bound? If not, how can I make it so? Can I make it SMARTER?

After I make it SMARTER, what next steps do I need to take to move toward achieving it?

What tools or resources do I need in order to achieve my goal? Does it require money? Equipment? Space? Assistance from people?

Who has already done what I'm trying to do? Would they be willing to advise me on how to best reach my goal? Is this a goal I can pursue with someone else to make it easier to reach?

Now, assign a specific deadline when each step needs to be completed.

When is the optimal time I can work on these steps?

Am I properly motivated? Do I have a system in place for reaching the goal over the long term?

Do I have a plan for when pursuit of the goal gets thrown off track? Do I know how I will handle or recover from interruptions, setbacks, or mistakes?

What does "done" look like? How will I know when I've completed my goal? You may think it's self-evident, but it's a good practice to state it explicitly so there are no surprises at the end.

We recommend writing the answers to these questions as they apply to exercise, fitness, and health. You can also write out how being fit and healthy will help you reach other life goals.

When you're finished answering the questions, you'll have a great blueprint for getting where you want to go.

TAKEAWAY: With a detailed blueprint in place, it becomes easier to reach your goals.

Putting It All Together

Repetition is the mother of learning,
the father of action, which makes it the architect
of accomplishment.

~ Zig Ziglar

There are really only two requirements when
it comes to exercise.
One is that you do it. The other is that
you continue to do it.

~ Jennie Brand-Miller

When it comes to exercise, fitness, and health, setting goals is a great thing. It's central to getting what you want. But there's one part of the plan that most people don't think about in advance.

Let's say you clarified your beliefs and priorities. You set goals that might stretch you a bit but they're definitely reachable. You got the right tools for the job and set off on your mission.

What happens after you've reached your goal? Do you go back to what you were doing before you started your exercise program? Do you set new goals? Do you simply continue along the same path?

After reaching their goal, many people simply go back to what they were doing before. One of the best examples of this is when people go on a diet. Countless people have gone on diets and lost weight, but relatively few have been able to keep the weight off for any length of time.

What about exercise? Unfortunately, many people decide to do it and then quickly lose interest. It's something to do for a short period of time until the novelty wears off or it becomes difficult.

It's clear that in order for the benefits of exercise, fitness, and health to be meaningful, structured programs have to become part of your life. Exercise and nutrition are not a temporary campaign for a short-term benefit.

When you were at the academy, you went through drill after drill and scenario after scenario. You learned that regular repetition is the key to success. It's how you learned your skills. And you also experienced over time the age-old truism: Use it or lose it.

This applies to exercise, fitness, and health as well. The tricky part is there's no final destination in the sense that you will be fit and healthy and then you can stop.

It's all about the journey and the process. With exercise, fitness, and health, the journey is the reward; being fit day in and day out is the goal.

The way people succeed in this endeavor is by putting together everything we discussed to this point:

- Understand your fears and what's holding you back.
- Develop the belief and create the vision of what you're trying to reach.
- Decide and commit as a sure way to succeed.
- Set your priorities.
- Establish SMART and SMARTER goals.
- Create a system to make reaching those goals easier.

When you put it all together, there is little that can stop you from reaching your goals.

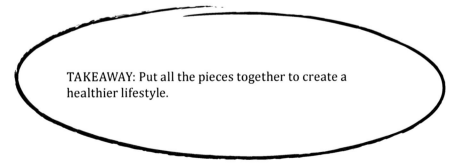

TAKEAWAY: Put all the pieces together to create a healthier lifestyle.

Lee Puts It All Together

Success is how high you bounce when you hit bottom.

~ George S. Patton

*Always be yourself, express yourself,
have faith in yourself. Do not go out and look for
a successful personality and duplicate it.*

~ Bruce Lee

They call him "Big Lee" and "Big Country." As you can imagine, these aren't the nicknames of a small fella.

Standing six feet two inches, Officer Stephenson hit the scales at 382 lbs. "It seems the one constant thing I have in my life is being overweight. Over time, I've had to buy clothes with an increasing number of Xs in front of the 'Large' when it came to size."

When he was 45 years old, Lee could no longer avoid his fear and pretend that all was ok. His wake-up call came in the form of a triple bypass with three arteries blocked at nearly 100 percent. As it turned out, it wasn't much of a wake-up call. "It lasted about a year, then I slowly slid back into my comfortable old habits of poor diet and sedentary lifestyle."

He got a complete physical exam and made a smart and brave decision: he spoke with his doctor about the depression and anxiety that surrounded his health issues. It was time to face his fear instead of just doing the superficial work of losing some weight.

"I got serious about taking the blood pressure and cholesterol meds that I'd been neglecting. Next, I adjusted my diet. Third, I got off the couch and started moving my body. And the doctor prescribed something for my depression and anxiety."

In that first month, he lost 25 lbs. by changing his diet and going to the gym almost every day. In the next two months, he lost another 22 lbs. "My cholesterol and everything else was in normal ranges."

He cut out all fast food, stopped eating out during work, and reduced the number of times he was going out to dinner each week. "My wife and I started cooking. We enjoy it because now we communicate about the healthy options we can create and we like spending time together."

"I carry a small cooler in my unit with my meal along with water and snacks like fruit, nuts, crackers, and cheese. I try to eat three small meals and three healthy snacks each day."

One of the biggest changes Lee has made is one we hear about from countless people: "I don't mindlessly eat to relieve stress anymore. When I get that feeling, I eat something healthy, do something around the house, or exercise to reduce the stress."

He's also been smart about portion sizes. "I use a smaller plate or bowl and give myself time before grabbing seconds or thirds. If I wait, I usually don't get seconds or thirds because my stomach has time to signal my brain that I don't need anymore."

More importantly, he examined his fears. He worried about how others saw him. He feared increased medical issues if he didn't make changes. And he was afraid of not being able to handle setbacks.

All of this has had a wonderful influence on his family. "My kids are excited and pleased to see their father finally making and maintaining positive changes in his health and lifestyle. My wife is excited too and very supportive of my endeavor. It has brought us closer together as we now communicate more.

For more details on Lee's workout, diet, and how he stays motivated, see Lee Stephenson's Path on p. 138

TAKEAWAY: Combine the information in this book for a multi-pronged approach to fitness and health.

Part 4

Components of Fitness

Lesson 23

Five Components of Physical Fitness

I really don't think I need buns of steel. I'd be happy with buns of cinnamon.

~ Ellen DeGeneres

Exercise is a dirty word. Every time I hear it, I wash my mouth out with chocolate.

~ Charles M. Schulz

There are five basic components of fitness: cardiovascular endurance, muscle strength, muscle endurance, flexibility, and body composition.

All have their own level of importance, but some may be more useful to you depending on your health and occupational needs.

Each of these components will be discussed individually in detail in the next few lessons. Generally speaking, exercise should target one or more of these five areas.

Many would agree that *cardiovascular endurance* is the most important component of exercise and should be given the highest priority.

However, when you're on patrol and get into a wrestling match with a 285-pound intoxicated bar patron, the thought that "maybe I should have lifted a few more weights" could possibly come to mind. And a left hamstring giving out while you're chasing a suspect can make you realize how you might not have been stretching as much as you should!

Why is it, then, that cardiovascular exercise is listed first? Perhaps this statistic will help: Approximately 40% of deaths in the United States are due to cardiovascular disease and stroke. Try to find how many deaths each year are from weak biceps or pulled hamstrings.

While all components will play a role in job performance, the long-term benefits of cardiovascular exercise will remain the most important factor in your fitness and health.

Weight training will bring increased *muscle strength* and *muscle endurance*. One way to differentiate the two is to compare a baseball pitcher and a hitter. The pitcher needs a great deal of muscle endurance to repeatedly throw the ball over the plate. The hitter relies on muscle strength to send the ball across the park one time.

The other somewhat unrealized benefit of weight training and adding muscle is that muscle is metabolically active tissue. This means that it takes about 35 calories per day just to maintain one pound of muscle. The bottom line is that the 2 lbs. of muscle you have added this year from weight training equals over 7 lbs. of fat burned per year.

Flexibility is the ability to move a joint through a range of motion. While this may not seem initially that important, your range of motion and ability to move freely dramatically decrease as you age. It's important to keep your flexibility as much as possible. Your flexibility is a key to other issues. For example, as you grow older and develop lower back pain, hamstring flexibility helps minimize that pain.

The final component of fitness is *body composition*. This term refers to the amount of body fat you have. Increased amount of body fat is linked to several metabolic diseases including heart disease, diabetes, and hypertension.

Body composition can be improved through a combination of cardiovascular exercise and proper nutrition.

While there is no one "best" exercise, certainly a well-rounded program should emphasize all the components of fitness.

TAKEAWAY: Let the five components work together to give you great fitness.

Lesson 24

Cardiovascular Endurance

*Most people never run far enough on their first wind
to find out they've got a second.*

~ William James

*Endurance is one of the most difficult disciplines,
but it is to the one who endures that
the final victory comes.*

~ Buddha

The most reliable measure of fitness is generally considered to be how well the human heart is working, commonly referred to as cardiovascular fitness.

"Cardio" means heart; the heart is an electrical-mechanical pump about the size of your fist. "Vascular" refers to the vessels that move your body's 5 liters of blood to and from the heart. Obviously, it's imperative that this small organ work properly all the time, both electrically and mechanically.

Electrical disturbances are generally referred to as "arrhythmias" and may cause short-circuits in the body's ability to pump blood. Some electrical disturbances can lead to mechanical problems, thereby decreasing or even stopping the flow of blood to the heart.

The heart needs a blood supply in order to work properly, and this is supplied by the coronary arteries. These particular blood vessels supply blood and oxygen solely to the heart, allowing the pump to do its job and deliver blood throughout the body.

Failure to take care of the heart with proper nutrition and exercise can result in the vessels becoming filled with fatty plaque build-up, decreasing blood flow to the heart, thereby increasing the risk of a heart attack or stroke.

Besides increased risk of heart attack or stroke, lack of cardiovascular fitness can lead to other problems, such as diabetes and hypertension.

The cardiopulmonary system includes the heart and lungs. The heart works with the lungs to ensure that the human body receives an adequate supply of oxygen. Decreased cardiovascular function can be associated with pulmonary (lung) issues as the interconnected nature of these two organs cannot be underestimated.

For quality of life as well as longevity, it's imperative to work on improving these vital organs of the body.

What is the most effective way to induce positive changes in the cardiovascular and the cardiopulmonary system?

The simplest and most direct answer is to move your body!

Inactivity will drastically decrease the function of the heart. In other words, your heart is like an engine — it wants to run, it wants to go. If you leave your car in the garage without starting it up for long periods of time, it will become sluggish and non-responsive. The same thing is true of the heart. Therefore, the best way to get the heart moving is for you to move!

Regular exercise has been shown to assist greatly with keeping the coronary vessels clean and blood flowing smoothly, thereby reducing the risk for cardiovascular problems.

Make sure you fully appreciate the value of these systems of the body. Often we take them for granted until something happens that has a drastic effect on our lives. Take a proactive approach in dealing with your heart — it will pay dividends for many years!

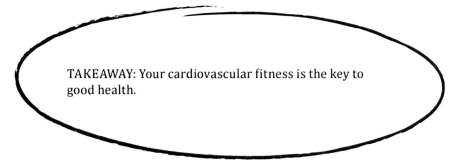

TAKEAWAY: Your cardiovascular fitness is the key to good health.

Muscle Strength

Practice puts brains in your muscles.

~ Sam Snead

It's not about weight, it's about fitness,
and one component of being fit
is to have relatively low body fat, because fat is
not very efficient, whereas muscle is.

~ Deborah Bull

Strength is defined as the ability of a muscle (or muscle groups) to produce force. The stronger individual muscles, the more force they can produce. Power is quite similar to strength, with a slight exception. Power is the ability to produce force in a short amount of time.

Muscle strength is extremely important from a fitness standpoint. The skeletal muscles are needed to produce force in order to produce movement or do any type of work. Increasing strength can provide the benefit of producing more force, which allows you to more easily perform functions requiring greater strength.

An increase in strength can also lead to increases in energy levels as well as a decreased risk of injury as stronger muscles are more resistant to outside forces.

From a health and fitness standpoint, muscle strength is extremely important for the prevention of certain conditions, primarily osteoporosis. Stronger muscles can also reduce the risk of cardiovascular disease, hypertension, and diabetes.

Skeletal muscle is metabolically active tissue, so an additional benefit of adding more muscle is the ability to burn extra calories even when you are not active. Therefore, strength training will also help improve your body composition levels.

To assess strength levels, many individuals utilize the One Repetition Maximum (1RM) assessment method. This involves lifting the maximum amount of weight you can possibly lift. However, caution is necessary when utilizing this as novice lifters or individuals with questionable technique have been known to suffer serious injuries.

A primary purpose of working out is generally to acquire strength and not to demonstrate it. Therefore, a strength assessment may not be needed.

What is the best way to increase muscle strength? A high-intensity resistance exercise program consisting of low repetitions with high resistance has been shown to be most effective in accomplishing strength gains.

Strength levels can be enhanced by utilizing either free weights, machines, or even body-weight exercises. Anything that provides resistance to the body can be effective in increasing strength levels. The key is properly overloading the muscles and keeping proper form and high intensity.

While the workout program is the most important component, proper nutrition and adequate rest are essential parts of increasing muscle strength. Without the proper nutrients to feed the working muscles, as well as adequate recovery time after the workout, muscle strength will be extremely difficult to achieve.

From a law enforcement perspective, strength is an essential component in order to perform the job effectively. From pushing a car to "dealing with" a suspect, strength is essential to this profession.

Muscle strength more than likely has an additional deterrent effect when dealing with individuals who might not want your company. Intuitively, individuals might think twice about confronting an officer who is physically imposing versus a smaller officer.

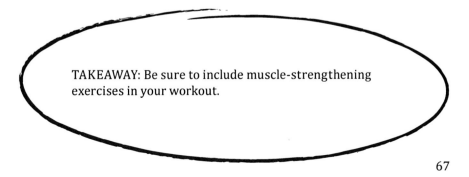

TAKEAWAY: Be sure to include muscle-strengthening exercises in your workout.

Lesson 26

Muscle Endurance

A feeble body weakens the mind.

~ Jean-Jacques Rousseau

15 minutes a day! Give me just this and
I'll prove I can make you a new man.

~ Charles Atlas

Muscle endurance is the ability of a muscle (or muscle groups) to repeatedly contract over time. The opposite of muscle endurance is muscle fatigue, or the inability of muscles to contract.

We generally think of muscle endurance when someone has to sustain an activity for a long period of time. Often the term "endurance" refers to activities such as marathons and races that demand a high degree of cardiovascular stamina.

However, even in those races, the heart muscle is not the only part of the body that has to keep contracting time after time. For example, in a marathon, the muscles of the lower extremities are asked to respond by producing force over and over again.

Benefits of increasing muscle endurance include a reduction in body fat and sustaining proper weight control. An additional benefit is increased energy and vitality.

Muscle endurance has also been shown to decrease stress levels as well as reduce anxiety and depression.

What do these benefits have to do with police work?

Perhaps a better question would be which of the benefits that muscle endurance offers doesn't apply to police work?

Think back in your career when you were in a situation that seemed to go on forever, like a standoff of some type. Have you been in a situation where the concept of muscle endurance suddenly became extremely important, such as a foot pursuit? A lengthy wrestling match with a suspect? Standing for hours on end while directing traffic?

It may be fairly easy to understand how muscle endurance is important in many of those situations, but more difficult to imagine how it's related to simply standing in place. Even though you are not moving, your muscles are still responsible for exerting force in order to hold your body weight steady.

To make things more difficult, don't forget to add in the few extra pounds of gear you're carrying. Muscle endurance now becomes extremely important.

Lack of endurance will lead to muscle fatigue and muscle fatigue will quickly take you out of the race — or the chase.

A strong piece of advice is not to wait until you experience a situation where you wished you had just a bit more muscle endurance. Spend some time increasing this invaluable component of fitness.

What is the best way to increase muscle endurance? A resistance exercise program should be used that focuses on strict form repetitions as opposed to higher-weight repetitions. In other words, if you're interested in endurance more than strength, decrease the amount of resistance in the resistance program and increase the number of repetitions.

For example, instead of one set of 8 repetitions with 80 lbs., perform two sets of 15 repetitions at 55-60 lbs.; increasing repetitions and decreasing resistance is the key to improving muscle endurance.

TAKEAWAY: Muscle endurance will help increase stamina and improve job performance.

Lesson 27
Flexibility

Take care of your body.
It's the only place you have to live.

~ Jim Rohn

Movement is a medicine for creating change in a
person's physical, emotional, and mental states.

~ Carol Welch

Most people dismiss the importance of flexibility because they tend to think of flexibility as gymnasts literally bending over backwards or martial artists kicking their leg straight up into the air. We view those images and wonder, "Why do I need to be that flexible?"

The truth is you don't need to get your leg up over your head.

"So, why do I need flexibility at all?"

The importance of flexibility begins with a definition. Flexibility is simply defined as range of motion. Range of motion is the ability to move a joint or facilitate articulation (two or more bones coming together) from its anatomical position to its extreme limit. Simply, it's how far you can move.

Why is range of motion important? Range of motion is necessary to perform everyday activities, either at home or on the job: to successfully and painlessly get out of your patrol car, get out of your chair, to reach your belt in order to remove your handcuffs or service weapon, and even to extend while wrestling with a suspect.

Flexibility is typically not thought of as important until it goes away. Research has shown that improved flexibility reduces the risk of injury during exercise and other activities.

The shape and contact area of your bones can impact your flexibility.

For example, when you extend your elbow, it generally can only go straight. The reason it does not go any further is because the shapes of the two bones articulating prevent it from moving any further.

The majority of your range of motion, however, relies on the extensibility of your muscles. The tighter the muscles, the less range of motion; the more extensible, or looser the muscles, the greater the range of motion.

How can you increase your flexibility? The only way to increase your flexibility is through proper stretching techniques. The less you stretch, the less flexible you will be. The important point to remember in a flexibility program is to "stretch, don't strain."

An overall stretching routine should only take about 5-7 minutes of your time. Research has shown that, for maximum benefit, a stretch should be held for about 15-20 seconds. In the case of stretching, more is not necessarily better: get into the stretched position and hold it for a quarter of a minute — don't bounce, don't jerk, just stay relaxed. The benefits will come your way!

Probably the one deeply underappreciated aspect of stretching is that improved flexibility can reduce stress in the working muscles and help release tension developed throughout the day. While both stress and tension are unique to each individual, a proper stretching program has been shown to assist in these areas.

For a minimum investment of about 5 minutes per day, three to four days a week, you can reduce your risk of lower back issues, reduce tension, reduce stress, and improve your ability to move.

TAKEAWAY: Stretching can strengthen your body and help prevent injury.

Lesson 28
Body Composition

It's simple: if it jiggles, it's fat.

~ Arnold Schwarzenegger

If you keep on eating unhealthy food then,
no matter how many weight loss tips you follow,
you are likely to retain weight and become obese.
If only you start eating healthy food, you will be
pleasantly surprised how easy it is to lose weight.

~ Subodh Gupta

One of the most important ways we can view the human body is by analyzing its composition. Many mechanisms work together to formulate body composition, including bones, muscles, internal organs, and skin.

From a health and fitness perspective, body composition typically refers to the amount of fat tissue present.

Some body fat is important for everyday living and to maintain the processes necessary for growth and reproduction. That's your "essential fat," which makes up about 3-5% of a male's body weight, and from 8-12% of a female's body weight. Females need more for childbearing and hormonal functions necessary to maintain life.

However, not all body fat is essential. Humans tend to store fat due to the excessive intake of calories. For police officers, this is sometimes a very easy thing to do!

The downside is that increased body fat has been linked to many diseases and other conditions, including heart disease, hypertension, diabetes, and several forms of cancer. Another negative to carrying around excess fat is that it creates additional stress on the bones and joints, making movement more difficult, with an increased risk of arthritis.

Fat does have some function in the body: It stores the fat soluble vitamins including Vitamin A, D, E and K. Fat tissue serves as a long-term energy source and also acts as insulation and protection.

The negatives, however, far outweigh the positives, especially when fat builds up around the midsection. Excessive fat in the abdominal area is linked to an increased risk of cardiovascular disease.

How do you change your body composition?

If you choose just to eat wisely and not exercise, you may lose body fat but you will not increase your muscle size. While that may be one way of accomplishing this goal, the addition of muscle to the body does have several important advantages, including strength and ease of movement.

If you choose just to exercise but not be careful with your nutrition, your fitness level may increase, but you will not be able to function at the level necessary for optimal performance. Also, even though your body is burning some calories through exercise, it may not be able to keep up with the increased calories, thereby resulting in increased fat storage.

The most promising solution is to combine both a well-designed exercise program and proper nutrition. These two will work together to help you achieve the changes you want to make in your body composition.

Not sure you understand why you need both? Try this as an example. Hop across the room on just one foot. Somewhat difficult, isn't it? Now try hopping across the room with just the other foot. That wasn't much easier, unfortunately. By using only one component of your body to accomplish a task, great results can be difficult to obtain. But what if you let both components work together to help achieve the goal?

TAKEAWAY: You can change your body composition through a balance of exercise and nutrition.

Problem Area I — Heart and Lungs

Exercise should be regarded as tribute to the heart.

~ Gene Tunney

*I could feel my anger dissipating as the miles went by
— you can't run and stay mad!*

~ Kathrine Switzer

People often use the words "cardiovascular" and "cardiopulmonary" synonymously. However, the cardiovascular system strictly refers to the heart and blood vessels; the cardiopulmonary system refers to the heart and lungs.

The importance of the heart and lungs working together is fully realized when either one of them doesn't do its share of the work.

As we mentioned, the heart, quite simply, is an electrical/mechanical pump. The basic purpose of this fist-sized apparatus is to propel blood carrying oxygen through your body and then return used blood back to the lungs. It is hopefully a process that doesn't end prematurely.

The process can become complicated when this complex piece of machinery doesn't work right. If the heart doesn't get the proper electrical signal sent through it or it becomes clogged, the pump will cease to work properly. And this is one pump that has severe consequences if it breaks down.

Heart disease is the number one cause of death in the United States, accounting for over 25% of all deaths. The importance of a strong, reliable heart cannot be overemphasized. From preventing an early exit from this life to improved job performance, the heart must be in good working order each and every day.

For police officers, it's especially important to keep this pump working at an optimal level. The requirements of the job dictate that it run smoothly all the time.

The lungs work to deliver oxygen to the working muscles via the blood. Take a deep, deep breath. Hold it for a second. Now gradually let it out. How did that feel? Was it difficult? Did you not get very much air on that inhale? Do you get winded easily performing simple, everyday activities? You may need to have your lungs checked to see if they're functioning correctly.

Although pulmonary disease is responsible for approximately 12% of deaths in the U.S., often the importance of the lungs is underestimated. This is another aspect of the body we do not fully appreciate until it stops working at an optimal level.

Many of the pulmonary problems that police officers experience can be attributed to smoking.

In the past, much of society accepted smoking and didn't really pay attention to the problems that it could create in the body.

Today, the health risks associated with smoking are better understood. However, because smoking is so addicting, it's a difficult habit for many to let go.

This is especially true for police officers. Due to the high stress, sometimes boring, sometimes exhilarating, long hours type of job, it's natural for officers to seek a stress release. Exercise certainly is an excellent way to relieve stress and is a great alternative to smoking.

Think of the operation of the heart and lungs as a synergistic relationship. The whole is greater than the sum of its parts. These two organs work together to make your body function more efficiently. Taking care of both is extremely important. Let them work well together and they will help you work better as well!

TAKEAWAY: Your heart and lungs need to work together in order to deliver optimal performance.

Lesson 30

Problem Area II — Lower Back

Don't pray for lighter burdens,
but for stronger backs.

~ Unknown

Never give up, for that is just the place and time that
the tide will turn.

~ Harriet Beecher Stowe

The simple fact is 80% of people in the United States will suffer from lower back pain at some point in their lives. This type of problem can range from minor aches from lifting something incorrectly to debilitating issues requiring life-changing surgery.

While the lower back is generally not associated with mortality issues, it certainly can be a game changer in your life when it is not working correctly.

Police officers are susceptible to lower back pain for several reasons.

Most of the jobs in law enforcement are largely sedentary; police officers (certain types of patrol as well as administrators) tend to sit for long periods of time. These long periods of inactivity can allow excess weight to creep on the belly.

Anatomically, when sitting, the hips stay in a flexed position for long periods of time. This position tends to tighten up the important hamstring muscles of the upper leg.

Tight hamstring muscles, in turn, can cause an "anterior pelvic tilt," pushing the hips forward, placing even more stress on the lower back area.

Tight hamstrings, more tilt. More tilt, more back problems. More back problems, hamstrings continue to tighten. You now have a continuous loop of this problem. Somehow you need to break this loop.

So, what's the solution? How can you keep from becoming one of those four out of five people who will have this condition? What can you do if you already are one of those four and want to get rid of this pain?

First, and most important, anyone who is overweight needs to shed excess weight around the midsection. The combination of proper nutrition and cardiovascular exercise to burn off extra calories is the most effective way to accomplish this task.

By making even slight adjustments in both nutrition and exercise, you can make significant changes in the midsection that will pay off in many ways.

Second, work on strengthening the core muscles of the body. They are the abdominals, the lower back, and the side muscles known as the obliques. A strong core will help support the spine, allowing it to absorb much of the forces it encounters on a daily basis.

All movements in the body originate from the core and move to the periphery. A strong core is a solid foundation.

Third, stretch those hamstrings, gluteal, and lower back muscles. A little bit of flexibility goes a long way to counter back pain issues.

Fourth, get up from your desk at least every hour to move your body, stretch your legs, and clear your head. Research shows that staying active, even in the simplest ways, is as important as exercising.

Finally, stay with the program! Results will not be achieved by implementing these suggestions only once or twice.

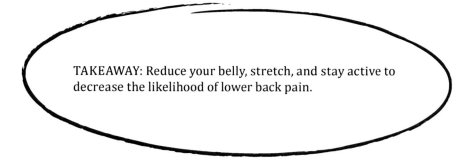

TAKEAWAY: Reduce your belly, stretch, and stay active to decrease the likelihood of lower back pain.

Part 5

Modalities

Modalities: What's Best and Why?

To keep the body in good health is a duty...
otherwise we shall not be able to keep our mind
strong and clear.

~ Buddha

The best thing you can do is the right thing;
the next best thing you can do is the wrong thing;
the worst thing you can do is nothing.

~ Theodore Roosevelt

Modality, or mode of exercise, means the type of exercise performed. Depending on individual needs, goals, and desires, the modality becomes an increasingly important part of your exercise program.

Cardiovascular exercise can be divided into three basic modalities: Non-weight-bearing, semi-weight-bearing, and full-weight-bearing.

Non-weight-bearing exercise means that the body is completely supported in some fashion. There are two ways of performing non-weight-bearing exercise. The first is to book a ticket to the space station and engage in an exercise program in zero gravity.

The other non-weight-bearing modality that may be a bit more realistic is swimming. The body is completely supported by the water. Equipment needs are minimal: A body of water, swimsuit, goggles, towel, and off you go.

While the advantage of this type of exercise is that it's very low stress on the joints, the disadvantage is that it's difficult to raise your heart rate and maintain it at a worthwhile level. Swimming is very much a skill sport, and typically beginners swim about a length of the pool and then stop to catch their breath.

Semi-weight-bearing exercise means that the body is partially supported in some fashion. Examples of this type of modality include bicycles, elliptical trainers, and some Stairmaster-type climbing machines.

The only disadvantage is that you need specialized equipment. However, most health clubs and fitness centers have various machines of this type. Many different home versions are available as well. The advantage of semi-weight-bearing exercise is that it's easy to start, easy to continue, and most types of this modality are still easy on the joints.

Full-weight-bearing exercise means the body is completely free from any outside support. Examples of this modality include walking, running, and many different group exercise classes including Step Aerobics.

The advantage of this type of exercise is that it is easy to perform, generally low cost (a good pair of shoes), and burns a great many calories. The disadvantage of full-weight-bearing exercise is that it's hard on the joints. The repetitive load, especially from running, puts a great deal of stress on multiple joints including the ankles, knees, and the lower back.

So, which one is best and why? While all of the types of exercises have advantages and disadvantages, care needs to be taken in choosing the correct modality according to your preference. The one that is best is the one that fits you best. In other words, which one do you enjoy doing and which one will you continue to do?

We may tell you that swimming is the "best" modality based on your individual needs and goals, but if you hate to swim, the probability of success is extremely low. An elliptical machine is a great modality for burning calories, but if you don't like to exercise indoors, this program will not last long.

Find the one you *want* to do. Exercise will only be effective if you stick to it. Don't get caught up in the science of this — the psychological part is much more important!

TAKEAWAY: Choose the modality that's most enjoyable to you so you'll keep exercising.

Lesson 32

Weight Training Basics: Form and Intensity

I consider my refusal to go to the gym today as resistance training.

~ Unknown

Training gives us an outlet for suppressed energies created by stress and thus tones the spirit just as exercise conditions the body.

~ Arnold Schwarzenegger

An important modality of exercise is resistance training, or weight training.

Resistance training has been used for many years in order to increase the strength of the working muscles. Surprisingly, it also has a positive effect on the heart muscle. Therefore, a proper weight-training program can offer many benefits with little investment of time.

Where to begin? There is so much information available on weight training that it's difficult to know where to start.

The most important piece of advice is to *begin gradually.* Many people begin weight-training programs and do too much too soon. They quit because they were too sore to continue. Successful weight training cannot happen overnight. Don't rush it!

Should you use free weights or machines? Which is better? The debate has raged on for years. The answer is simple: which one can you perform safely and which one do you enjoy doing?

As far as the myth goes that free weights will "bulk" you up and machines will "tone" you, we offer this: the contracting muscle only knows that it is being called upon to produce force against a resistance — and with that stimulation, proper hormones, nutrients, and adequate rest, the muscle will grow.

Without all of those variables in place, you will not achieve muscle growth. Simply put, if you contract a muscle (or muscles) against a proper resistance, it will respond!

"Well, how come my buddy has 20-inch biceps and I only have 13, but I work harder than he does?"

Much of your potential for muscle growth is derived from your genetic makeup — you may inherit your potential for muscle growth from your parents. Weight training can help you get to your potential, whatever that may be.

Focus on weight training should be on the two most important principles: Form and intensity. After this, most everything will fall into place.

Form simply means doing everything you possibly can to isolate the muscle group you are working. Proper form is important to ensure that the muscle you want to have working *is* the muscle that is working. By compromising your form, you risk more than just lack of results; quite often poor form can lead to injuries, both minor and severe.

Intensity is referred to how hard you exercise, or how far you will go.

Generally, you can think of a set of 12 repetitions as two parts: the first 10 repetitions and the last two. In other words, the last two repetitions will give you as much benefit as the first 10.

Too often you stop exercising when your mind tells you to stop and not when your muscles tell you to stop. Your mind will quit long before your body will.

Developing that drive to keep going (while maintaining proper form) will offer the best avenue to achieve great results from your weight-training program.

TAKEAWAY: Without proper form and intensity, you will just be wasting your time in the weight room.

Lesson 33

Weight Training Basics: Sets and Reps

*Sore muscles are nothing compared to
the pain of regret.*

~ Toni Sorenson

*The last three or four reps is what makes the
muscle grow. This area of pain divides the champion
from someone else who is not a champion.*

~ Arnold Schwarzenegger

The two most important principles in weight training are form and intensity. However, in order to have an effective program, other basic principles should be followed.

How many exercises should you do? Depending on individual desires and limitations, a basic program should be about 4-6 lower body exercises and 6-8 upper body exercises in each workout.

This equates to about 12 different exercises in a single session. This will form the basis of a good overall routine that will not take too much time and still be effective in gaining strength.

How many sets? When beginning a program, only one set should be performed, minimizing possible muscle soreness and potential for injury. You can increase the number of sets later.

How many repetitions in each set? If your goal is muscle endurance, keep the amount of weight low and the repetitions high, around 12-15 or more. If you're interested in greater strength gains, keep the weight high and your repetitions low (about 4-6). If you want somewhere in between those two, keep the repetitions in each set between 8 and 12.

What is the optimal order of the exercises? The best order of exercises is generally working from your largest muscle groups down to your smallest groups.

Large groups include the gluteus maximus (butt), quadriceps and hamstrings in the lower body, and the pectoralis major (chest) and latissimus dorsi (upper back) in the upper body. Smaller groups would be the triceps, biceps, and calves.

The reason you begin with larger groups is twofold: First, larger muscles will stimulate more growth throughout the body — the larger the muscle group, the greater the effect on the rest of the body. Second, some of your smaller muscle groups serve as "links" between your large groups and some exercises.

For example, if you work out your biceps before you do back work, your back exercises will not be as effective because the biceps act as helper muscles in many latissimus exercises and now they're fatigued.

How often should I lift? Skeletal muscle is not the same as your cardiac (heart) muscle. While you can work your heart every day and still see improvement, your skeletal muscles need a bit more rest. The recommendation is to wait at least 48 hours in between workouts for the muscles to recover.

If you must go to the gym six days a week, split up your body parts something like this: chest, shoulders, and triceps on one day; legs, back, and biceps the next. This will allow you the 48 hours of rest between body parts.

Start with the basics of form and intensity, then develop a solid program based on number of exercises, sets, repetition, and the proper order. Most importantly, weight training by nature is repetitious. Establish a program you can do on a consistent basis for best results!

TAKEAWAY: Allow the large muscle groups to have a positive effect on the rest of the body.

Lesson 34

Other Modalities of Exercise

I'm not telling you it's going to be easy, I'm telling you it's going to be worth it.

~ Art Williams

*Ability is what you're capable of doing.
Motivation determines what you do.
Attitude determines how well you do it.*

~ Lou Holtz

In fitness and health, the basics will always remain the basics. You can go a long way by focusing on the fundamentals of exercise and nutrition in order to have the fitness and health you want.

But at some point your interest may turn to other, more complex aspects of fitness. You might like to enter a running competition or complete an extremely long bicycle ride. Or pursue one of the many different athletic endeavors and contests that seem to have sprung up lately.

Deciding to participate in such activities can be very helpful in maintaining and improving fitness levels, and the successful completion of that goal makes all of that blood, sweat, and tears worthwhile.

All you have to do is look around a bit.

Besides the usual 5K races, 10K races, half marathons, and marathon runs, events including the Police Olympics have added a new dimension to competition.

The emergence and increased popularity of endurance competitions such as Muddy Buddys (Tough Mudders), Gladiator and Spartan contests, Adventure Races, and benefit bicycle rides have turned even couch potatoes into aspiring competitive athletes.

Different methods of physical training have also evolved into competitive opportunities. Crossfit has evolved from a method of training to its own competitions, now complete with prize money and television coverage.

Boot camps, while originally designed for training the military, have been introduced to the "civilian population." This may involve former military personnel as instructors to include some of the reality and harshness of what our troops actually have to go through, both physically and mentally.

Home video workouts have been popular for decades. These videos offer the opportunity to work out in the comfort of your own home, without the additional pressure of having anyone around to critique your performance.

Videos range from "boot camp" type activities, to cardiovascular exercises, and even yoga and other stretching type activities. Increasingly, home videos are available in a streaming format through your television, computer, and phone.

Which modality is the best? Once again it comes down to what you will enjoy doing in the long run. But we also need to keep in mind the safety issue. Along with the increased popularity of high-intensity workouts comes an increased incidence of muscle soreness and damage.

Individuals quite often have a tendency to do too much, too soon and end up experiencing problems resulting from these programs, leading to decreased enthusiasm for exercise in general. Many injuries occur from using improper form, so it is imperative to have adequate and proper instruction on all aspects of the planned exercise program.

Remember, the best way to begin is to make sure you start slowly, and keep in mind the safety precautions associated with each type of activity. Stay in this for the long run!

TAKEAWAY: Various exercise opportunities exist. Find the ones that will benefit you the most.

Part 6

Feeding Your Body

Nutrition

*Today, more than 95% of all chronic disease is
caused by food choice,
toxic food ingredients, nutritional deficiencies, and
lack of physical exercise.*

~ Mike Adams

*Every living cell in your body is made from
the food you eat. If you consistently eat junk food
then you'll have a junk body.*

~ Jeanette Jenkins

Nutrition is the largely unappreciated aspect of fitness. Many believe that if they simply work out on a regular basis, it will suffice for becoming fit and "in shape."

But, like a car, the body needs the right fuel to operate properly. The fuel that supplies you had better be of high quality or you'll find yourself running inefficiently at best.

Police work, however, tends to make eating properly a difficult task, and, as a result, many officers quickly add unwanted pounds.

Many people turn to a diet when they wish to lose weight. However, this may not always be the best approach to solving the weight problem. There are many diets that proclaim to be the best in order to help you lose weight. Or get stronger. Or look better. Or tone you up.

Many diets make false claims, and some are potentially dangerous.

A great recommendation is to take the term "diet" out of your vocabulary and replace it with "nourishment," "nutrition," and "lifestyle." The word diet implies "temporary." A diet is a temporary way to lose weight.

And when you lose the weight you desire and go back to eating the way you did before, you gain that weight back (and usually more). Therefore, it's extremely important to make changes in your nutrition and lifestyle that are reasonable and long term.

What are some reasonable and practical applications you can introduce into your nutrition program?

1. Don't be too afraid of fast food — but make a couple of modifications. The grilled chicken sandwich is a healthy alternative. Go with grilled instead of fried.

2. Eliminate French fries or tater tots at your meals.

3. Don't turn a salad into a caloric monster; be careful of the toppings and the dressings that add a lot of calories.

4. Long day? Ready to eat some "comfort food"? Before you give in, replace the comfort foods with a little activity. You will be surprised at how good it feels NOT to eat something that isn't good for you.

5. Don't forget to eat breakfast — it's the most important meal of the day. And make sure you add a protein source to maintain your energy throughout the morning.

6. Don't starve yourself! You can only lose approximately 2 lbs. of fat per week. This is a long-term process — take it slow and steady!

7. Want to gain some weight? Largely focus on your resistance exercise — you will need some extra calories, but make sure they are the healthy kind.

8. Late night hunger pains? Instead of eating, brush your teeth or drink some water. You will be amazed at what these simple acts will do to your appetite!

The foundation of activity, performance, and weight control lies in proper nutrition. Proper nutrition has long-term benefits; unfortunately poor nourishment has long-term consequences!

TAKEAWAY: A "diet" lifestyle will add pounds to your waist; a nutritious lifestyle will help you keep fit.

Lesson 36

Portion Control

*Your life does not get better by chance,
it gets better by change.*

~ Jim Rohn

*If you don't do what's best for your body, you're the
one who comes up on the short end.*

~ Julius Erving

A fundamental concept in proper nutrition habits is portion control. Portion control is an easy concept to understand but a difficult one to master.

We live in a society that seems to embrace overconsumption, especially when it comes to food. We have made it quite easy to eat too much with the all-you-can-eat buffets, super-sizing meals, adding chips and a drink, and other ways restaurants work to increase their business.

We also love to overindulge. As you know, in some ways, this becomes an even bigger challenge for law enforcement. We concerned citizens of the community like nothing more than to bring our beloved officers cookies and cakes on special occasions, like Christmas, Thanksgiving, the 4th of July, and pretty much any other holiday on the calendar.

Then there are the fundraisers, cookouts, parties, and any other number of ways to eat and drink our way to bad health.

Portion control will continue to be one of the biggest challenges facing officers. It's important to embrace the idea that "more is not necessarily better" and implement it in your daily habits.

Many solutions have been proposed to tackle portion control such as using smaller plates at your meal times, eating smaller portions more frequently throughout the day, or drinking a full glass of water before you eat.

People use reward days as a way to satisfy their need for overconsumption and overindulgence. While this can be successful, quite often the reward day turns into two days, two days goes to three, and before long you're right back where you were in the first place.

These approaches can be effective in your nutrition "battle," but a key concept in your struggle with portion control is discipline. Once again, we have said something that seems fairly simplistic on its face, but extremely difficult to implement on a daily basis.

Self-discipline is the ability to control one's feelings and overcome individual weaknesses as well as the ability to pursue what you think is right despite temptations.

What weaknesses could you possibly have with your diet? What about the temptation of taking an extra piece of cake at your partner's birthday party? Or ordering the large fries with the meal because you're working a double? Or that extra scoop of ice cream after a particularly long day in court?

Self-discipline needs to be embraced as an integral part of your daily battle with food portions. Enlist your family and friends in your effort to exercise, get fit, and be healthy.

Many good quotations are associated with self-discipline, but this one seems appropriate for your battle with portion control: "Discipline is choosing between what you want NOW and what you want MOST."

Sure, that piece of cake would taste good NOW. But, if you truly want to reduce your waist size or impress your cardiologist, maybe that cake doesn't seem all that appealing. Or the extra ice cream that tomorrow you really won't remember anyway.

What do you want MOST?

TAKEAWAY: Use simple techniques to bring your portion size under control.

Lesson 37

Hydration

Water is the driving force of all nature.

~ Leonardo da Vinci

*Thousands have lived without love,
not one without water.*

~ W. H. Auden

Any discussion of exercise, fitness, and health would not be complete without including something about hydration.

The body can live for over three weeks without food; however, it can live less than one week without water. Many of us take hydration for granted. "I drink enough water. I take sips from the water fountain all day...."

Most of us don't get enough fluids in our bodies on a regular basis. Very few officers properly hydrate, made worse by long hours of perspiring in hot uniforms and carrying extra gear.

What is the solution to the problem of dehydration? The answer is simple: Hydrate! But what would be the best fluid replacement for you either on duty, off duty, or during or after your workout?

Water: Water is one of the essential nutrients of the body. "Essential" means that it is critical to life. If you've been perspiring a lot, be sure to replace that lost water. Start your day with a glass of water to wake up your organs and replace lost water due to perspiration overnight.

The popular claim that you should drink 8-ounce glasses of water 8 times a day is not based on science and can be bad for you. Worried about drinking too much and adding extra weight? Water has no calories, so it will not add fat weight or produce energy.

Sports Drinks: These types of drinks, like Gatorade or Powerade, are a great way to get fluids back into the body as well as replacing lost electrolytes from perspiration after extreme exercise. However, they do contain calories and sugar. Generally, if you're active and are perspiring a great deal, these drinks would be a good choice in moderation.

Coffee/Soft Drinks: Coffee is a staple in your world and you may not be able to imagine life without it, but keep in mind that it contributes to your stress, fatigue, and negative moods. Soft drinks are high-sugar drinks with significant calories and all kinds of chemicals. Call them diet, call them caffeine-free. It doesn't matter. They in no way contribute to fitness and health.

Energy Drinks: These are calories in a bottle with a kick to keep you awake and frequently result in a significant impact after the high wears off. Extreme use of these drinks has been shown to be harmful. It's best to stay away from them altogether.

Milk: Milk is generally a good beverage, provided you are not lactose intolerant. It has calories, but this can be minimized by using skim or low fat milk. Chocolate milk is a preferred beverage for many after a workout as the combination of carbohydrates and protein makes for an ideal recovery drink.

Alcohol: All alcohol contains calories, with very little nutritional benefit. While we may drink alcohol for other reasons, it is not advisable to include it in your workout regimen. Evidence does exist that alcohol in moderation, particularly red wine, assists in the prevention of heart disease. Remember, the key word here is "moderation."

Is there a best beverage? When in doubt, drink water. Watch the calories. Be careful with the caffeine. Stay hydrated out there.

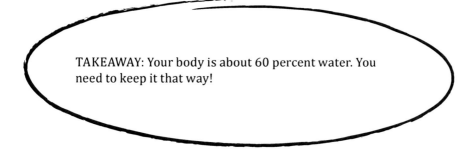

TAKEAWAY: Your body is about 60 percent water. You need to keep it that way!

Lesson 38

Vitamins and Supplements

The groundwork of all happiness is health.

~ Leigh Hunt

*It is health that is real wealth and not
pieces of gold and silver.*

~ Mahatma Gandhi

Vitamins are organic compounds that are essential for normal growth and development in the body. They're required to be consumed because they cannot be manufactured in the body.

They can be classified into water soluble and fat soluble. Water soluble vitamins that cannot be stored in the body are Vitamins B and C. These are eliminated by the body if taken in excessive amounts.

Fat soluble vitamins are Vitamins A, D, E and K; these are stored in the body in the adipose (fat) tissue. Because fat soluble vitamins can be stored for long periods of time, they can reach damaging or even toxic levels in the body if consumed in overabundance.

To dispel one myth, as vitamins do not contain calories, they cannot supply the body with energy. The only materials that can provide energy to the body are carbohydrates, fats, proteins, and alcohol, because all of those contain calories. However, vitamins assist the body in metabolizing those fuels into useable energy.

That Vitamin B12 shot that your partner recommended to increase your energy level? It will not give you additional energy (maybe it will if you think it will; don't underestimate the power of the placebo effect), but it may help convert suitable foods into useful energy.

An important consideration with vitamins is to understand that consumption does not necessarily equal absorption. Various factors may interfere with the body's ability to utilize vitamins, including age, gender, weight, smoking habits, and even how the vitamin is consumed. Also, certain medications may interfere with the body's ability to absorb vitamins.

Vitamin usage should be discussed with your physician to determine exactly what you require. Many individuals take a multi-vitamin which has many different vitamins and minerals combined into one tablet.

Two general recommendations include:

1. The multi-vitamin consumed should not exceed 100% of the Recommended Daily Allowance (RDA) as established by the Food and Nutrition Board for each vitamin.

2. Most men will not need a vitamin supplement that contains iron; too much iron has been linked to cardiovascular issues.

By definition a supplement is any substance not regularly consumed by the body utilized to enhance the body's performance. Some are legal, some are not; some will help you, some will not. The key lies in understanding the body and, more importantly, understanding what the supplement actually is. Supplements may include protein powders, pre-workout mixtures, and weight-gain formulas.

A key aspect in understanding supplements lies in the word itself: it is meant to *supplement* what you eat, not replace it. Most experts agree that it's best to get the bulk of nutrition from food. In this busy day and age — and considering the difficulties of eating correctly due to shift work — supplementation may be a good idea.

However, be careful taking supplements, especially if you are on any kind of medication. Drug-nutrient interactions can potentially have devastating consequences. Always seek the advice of your physician and a competent nutritional expert before consuming any type of vitamins or supplements.

TAKEAWAY: Vitamins and supplements can enhance body performance when taken correctly.

Part 7

Get Going

Lesson 39
Start Moving Toward Exercise

The secret of getting ahead is getting started.

~ Mark Twain

A man's health can be judged by which he takes two at a time — pills or stairs.

~ Joan Welsh

It's possible you haven't been in any kind of structured exercise routine in quite some time. That's fine. There's always a starting point for everything.

Instead of diving into a full-blown exercise routine that you'll quit after a couple of weeks, it may be best to start by understanding your starting point right now.

How active are you in your job and your daily life? Perform a "physical inventory" and calculate how much activity you are getting in your average day. This is a good time to face the brutal facts.

Do you go for walks with your spouse, family members, or friends? Even this modest movement is useful.

Do you park your car at the far end of the parking lot and walk to your office? This seemingly insignificant gesture has far greater positive effects than you might expect.

Do you play golf on your time off and walk the course? That makes a significant difference over riding in the golf cart through your 18 holes.

Do you have some land where you work cutting trees, hauling brush and hay, or building sheds? If so, your activity level is fairly high and it will burn a few calories.

Consider this: Matt's wife took a job at a local hospital as a dietitian. She soon dropped from 145 lbs. to 125, with her body fat decreasing as well. How did that happen? Simple: The hospital was three stories tall and she saw patients on each floor. Instead of taking the elevator, she walked the stairs *every time* she visited patients. Combined with a greater appreciation of proper nutrition, she was able to drop the weight and look and feel better!

While relatively unstructured activity is not a substitute for exercise, it's a great place to begin moving your body, especially if you find it necessary to ease into an exercise regimen, whether for physical reasons or reasons of willpower.

Keep in mind that you have chosen a profession that at times requires extreme physical agility and stamina. And it regularly inflicts mental stress. You don't know when that agility and stamina will be called on.

Start increasing your level of activity so you can move toward a regular exercise routine. This will help relieve much of the physical and mental stress of your job and give you more energy.

As you start increasing your activity, think about the transition to exercise by answering one simple question: What do you want to accomplish?

If you want to increase your fitness level and lose some weight, then the answer is you need an exercise program. If you want to get stronger or more flexible, the quickest way is through exercise. If you want to never contract a disease and remain healthy, live to be 110, and always enjoy your life, well....

No one can guarantee that you will not contract cancer or die of heart disease. No one can guarantee you that you will not become a diabetic. No one can guarantee that your blood pressure will not steadily rise as you age.

But research is definitive that exercise can decrease your risk for those conditions. Why not take a chance, overcome your fear, and increase your probability of a longer and healthier life?

TAKEAWAY: Increase your activity and start moving gradually to an exercise program.

Lesson 40

Beginning a Program Safely

Good seasons start with good beginnings.

~ Sparky Anderson

*The beginning is the most important part
of the work.*

~ Plato

The priorities of any exercise program are simple: safe, effective, fun.

Right now we need to focus on being safe. As you begin a program, there are a few precautions to take to make sure that it's safe and appropriate for you.

Most importantly, if you are a male over the age of 45 or a female over the age of 50, it's wise to check with your physician before beginning an exercise program.

Once your doctor says it's ok, here are some ideas to help get you started.

If you haven't done so up to this point, now is a good time to ask yourself, "Why am I attempting this program? What do I want to accomplish by working out or becoming more active?"

When you know what you want to accomplish, you'll know where to begin.

If you want to get active and trim down a bit, start with a slow walk and adjust your eating habits.

If you want to tone up, start with a light weight-lifting regimen.

If you're focusing on cardio health, jogging may be in the cards for you.

Establish your motivation and visualize your results. Without a firm understanding and appreciation of what you're getting yourself into, your chances of success are limited. If you have never experienced the benefits of physical fitness, you will have a limited appreciation of what a good program can do for you.

A key component in beginning an exercise program rests in these two words: "Start gradually."

This cannot be emphasized enough as many exercise programs have been scrapped because of excessive soreness or an early injury. You will actually make more progress starting slowly and gradually than you will if you push yourself too hard and get sidelined by an injury.

Unfortunately, initial excitement means you'll probably be impatient. Fight this urge and take your time. For example, it's ok to take one lap around the block every day for the first week or two. You may not feel like you've done anything or even break a sweat, but that's ok.

You also may soon experience the drudgery of repetition. You may quickly bore of the same walking route or repetitions in the weight room. You can change up your approach to your workout to keep your mind interested.

Finally, consult with people who know what they're talking about when it comes to physical fitness. Just because your buddy at work has 21-inch biceps doesn't necessarily mean he knows what's best for you; he may not understand your goals or your limitations.

Some people get great results *in spite of* what they did and not *because of* what they did! Most of us will find that if we do our research and work toward the goals, the benefits of the program will appear.

Yes, exercise is a science, and we need to be a little scientific if we want to reap the benefits. Do the research. You will benefit from the experience!

TAKEAWAY: Know what you're trying to accomplish and start slowly. Being safe is critical in an exercise program.

Make Your Workout Effective

*The main thing is to keep the main thing
the main thing.*

~ Stephen Covey

*To increase your effectiveness, make your emotions
subordinate to your commitments.*

~ Brian Koslow

If you're going to spend time in an exercise program, make sure it's effective.

Effectiveness essentially means "doing what you are supposed to be doing in the best way possible." Setting your goals and reaching them involves having an effective plan of achievement.

Your exercises should be performed with the idea that the program will produce the desired results. Remember not to beat yourself up if you don't reach your results once in a while. But, generally speaking, you should be going for results; otherwise, it's simply a waste of time, and you can't afford to use your time poorly.

Doing exercises you aren't sure about, whose purpose you don't understand, or don't know the correct way to do them undermines the effectiveness of your workout. Beyond that, performing those exercises can also be unsafe, causing injury to your body or bringing harm to those around you.

Seek out a trainer who has some experience in exercise development, but, more importantly, has the proper education and certifications in exercise program design.

Unfortunately, once in a while personal trainers will show clients exercises that the trainer personally likes, but aren't necessarily best suited for the individual's fitness level and goals.

Many people turn to the internet and questionable advertisements for advice on exercise and ways to achieve great results. There are so many products on the market that advertise a "quick fix," or "instant results." These products might promise to "melt the fat away," or "add 10 lbs. of solid muscle in 10 days!"

While these messages may look extremely promising, the truth is many of these products are simply gimmicks to make sure that a fool and his money are soon parted.

Another downside of such products is that they can be dangerous. For example, many diet aids are simply central nervous system stimulants, potentially causing rapid heart rates and cardiovascular complications. Stick with reputable, mainstream magazines and websites on exercise and fitness.

Keep in mind one of the major ways a gym setting can impact the effectiveness of your workout: socializing.

Most exercise professionals fully appreciate the value of going to the gym as a social endeavor; people join health clubs for a wide variety of reasons, only one of which is to get in shape.

They also know that one of the biggest dangers of going to a gym is losing focus. Often, the social aspects of a gym can outweigh the purpose of the workout, costing time and money, and creating distractions. This will have an impact on the effectiveness of the workout.

Understand what is important to you in your daily life. Make the most of your time in the gym, at home, or at work and be effective in your program. Wherever you work out, have a purpose and a goal in mind.

TAKEAWAY: Focus on the task at hand and perform the exercises in the correct way for best results.

Have Fun in Your Workout

*People rarely succeed unless they have fun in what
they are doing.*

~ Dale Carnegie

*Fitness needs to be perceived as fun and games or
we subconsciously avoid it.*

~ Alan Thicke

An exercise program, first and foremost, should be safe. Once that requirement is met, then the program should be effective. The third priority of an exercise program is that it should, at some point, be fun.

Often in life you can get into routines that become tedious. Exercise is no different.

In weight training, we speak of "sets" and "repetitions." These are called "repetitions" for a reason — a weight lifter must perform them over and over again. Exercise, by its very nature, is an activity that involves performing the same activity over and over again.

And some people thrive on the routine of doing the same thing over and over again. In exercise this can be an advantage.

Even though we use the term "routine," your exercise program does not have to become so mundane and predictable that you no longer enjoy it.

Enjoying an activity is of paramount importance in order to maintain interest; otherwise, chances are good that you won't stay with exercise in general.

What can you do to change up your workout and keep it fun?

- First, take a group exercise class, a spin class, try out a boot camp workout, join a run club, exercise with other people, use a video, make a game or challenge out of your exercise session.

- Second, get a personal trainer, go for a walk, or exercise in front of your favorite TV show. Just remember to take it slow and build up to it.

Your enjoyment level will increase as your fitness level increases.

If you simply don't enjoy exercising, it will be difficult to continue. Many people begin exercise programs because they have been forced into it (doctor's recommendation, significant other's urging, or other important reason).

It really doesn't matter what the reason. If you can't build some enjoyment into the program, chances are slim that you will stay with it for any length of time.

Matt is often asked, "What is the best exercise to do?" His answer is always: "What do you enjoy doing?"

For example, he could recommend that because you are overweight and suffer from osteoarthritis, swimming would be the best form of exercise for you. If your answer is, "I hate to swim," what are the chances you will stay with that program? Minimal.

There is a delicate balance between what is best for you and what you enjoy best. With some luck, those two will be the same. Keep the priorities of a program always close to you at all times.

Enjoy your workouts and have some fun!

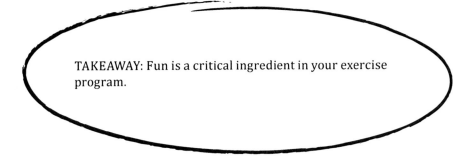

TAKEAWAY: Fun is a critical ingredient in your exercise program.

Lesson 43

Pain vs. Discomfort

Get comfortable with being uncomfortable!

~ Jillian Michaels

*I hated every minute of training, but I said,
"Don't quit. Suffer now and live the rest of
your life as a champion."*

~ Muhammad Ali

One of the most intriguing attitudes toward exercise is the belief that you have to suffer in order to get in shape. This alone has probably done more to drive people away from exercise than all other factors combined.

Most everyone starts with good intentions, but then they may experience some degree of muscle soreness or damage. This has the unwanted effect of decreasing their fondness for the activity.

You've probably heard the phrase associated with exercise, "No pain, no gain." We've seen it on t-shirts and heard it uttered in the gym. This is one of the most common sayings in the exercise world. Conventional wisdom is if you want to get bigger, stronger, or faster, you are going to have to suffer. And suffer a lot.

Let's explore this one a bit.

Pain is defined as physical suffering caused by illness or injury. This generally refers to the body being negatively impacted in some form or fashion. Pain is a good indication that something is wrong with the body.

We are now seeing that the results of heavy exercise are actually detrimental to the body. Studies show that marathon running can cause some damage to the heart. Individuals who engage in those types of activities may be going past the discomfort stage into the pain stage.

Let's just agree to get the idea that you have to suffer in order to improve out of your mind for a minute. "No pain, no gain" does not have a place in your exercise program.

Part of the problem is that if you're expecting it to be painful, you greatly reduce the probability that you'll ever start an exercise program.

And if you pursue an exercise program believing in "no pain, no gain," chances are good that you will hurt yourself.

Even if we reject the pain part of exercise, there is one thing we can guarantee: you will have to get out of your comfort zone in order to improve your current situation.

There's no way around it. All change, growth, and maturity happen when people decide to get out of their comfort zone, when they decide to do something they've never done before.

Your comfort zone is you sitting quietly, watching TV, eating a pizza. There's nothing wrong with that in itself. The problem arises when you do that but you know you should be doing something else, namely, exercising.

Instead of the pizza and TV, you have to reach for your sneakers, put them on, and get out of the house. Typically, there's nothing physically painful about this in the sense of "no pain, no gain," but it is uncomfortable.

When you get comfortable being uncomfortable, you will change your life. Instead of "no pain, no gain," think in terms of "effort in, results out."

TAKEAWAY: Forget about pain and choose discomfort. That's when you'll see great progress.

Lesson 44

Frequency of Exercise

*If it weren't for the fact that the TV set and the
refrigerator are so far apart,
some of us wouldn't get any exercise at all.*

~ Joey Adams

*Inaction breeds doubt and fear. Action breeds
confidence and courage. If you want to
conquer fear, do not sit home and think about it. Go
out and get busy.*

~ Dale Carnegie

There are many important considerations when beginning or continuing an exercise program. One variable is how many times per week to exercise.

There are 7 days in every week; therefore, the continuum of activity will range from 0-7 on frequency of exercise.

If you don't exercise at all — 0 days a week — you fall into a category called "inactive." This is the lack of purposeful exercise. No health benefit will be gained from inactivity and you have at least one major risk factor for cardiovascular disease.

If you exercise 1-2 days a week, you are a "recreational exerciser." Your reason for exercising is basically that someone talked you into it. "Hey, let's go to the gym and try Crossfit" or "Let's play softball this Friday." The benefit for this group is largely social.

When you exercise 2-3 days a week, you're exercising for health reasons. You're decreasing your risk of heart disease, decreasing your blood pressure, decreasing your risk of diabetes, and also reducing your risk of several forms of cancer. Working out 2-3 days a week will be helpful in beginning to see the benefits of a well-designed exercise program.

By participating 3-5 days a week, you're exercising to improve your fitness level. In addition to receiving health benefits, some other payoffs will begin to manifest themselves: you'll begin to lose some body fat and/or gain some muscle. Your overall physical conditioning will improve through greater heart and lung efficiency. You'll look and feel better.

If you participate 5-6 days a week, you're exercising for competitive reasons. While getting involved in competition is not necessarily the goal, this level of activity is generally associated with some type of fitness contest: a 10K race, a Muddy Buddy, or other competitive event.

If you work out 7 days a week with no break, this is called "exercise obsession." Too much of a good thing can turn into a bad thing.

Unfortunately, you can be addicted to exercise just as you can become addicted to alcohol or drugs. This obsessive level of exercise can lead to eating disorders and other illnesses. The body needs rest in order to heal. Taking at least one day off per week enables both the body and the mind to recover and to rejuvenate.

So, what is the optimal number of days per week to work out? That depends on what you're trying to accomplish.

0 and 7 are not good numbers as these represent the extremes. Recreation is fun but the health benefits will not be fully realized. You want health benefits? Attempt 2-3 sessions a week. Want to drop a few pounds? Better be working out at least 3-4 times. You want to compete? Shoot for 5 days a week.

Many factors will influence your frequency of exercise: shift work, family schedules, and availability of resources, among others. But, ultimately, you can set a schedule that will help you receive the benefits of your hard work.

TAKEAWAY: The number of times a week you exercise is directly related to the results you will achieve.

Intensity of Exercise

*I have to exercise in the morning before my brain
figures out what I'm doing.*

~ Marsha Doble

*The only exercise some people get is jumping to
conclusions, running down their friends,
side-stepping responsibility, and pushing their luck!*

~ Unknown

There are two basic methods to determine intensity of exercise: quantitative and qualitative.

Quantitative has to do with numbers. In this case, we'll use a percentage of your heart rate to determine the optimal range. You will need to know your Resting Heart Rate (RHR) in order to determine this figure.

Your RHR is most accurately taken after you wake up, get up, and then sit still for a short period (before you drink your coffee).

Place the tips of your second and third fingers on your opposite wrist on a line running down from the thumb. You should be able to feel your pulse at that point. Count the number of beats that occur in 15 seconds and multiply it by four. This is your Resting Heart Rate.

Now, subtract your age from 220. This is your Maximum Heart Rate (MHR), theoretically the maximum number of beats per minute your heart can contract. Subtract your Resting Heart Rate from your Maximum Heart Rate. This gives you a figure known as your Heart Rate Reserve (HRR).

Multiply your Heart Rate Reserve by .6. Add your Resting Heart Rate back to that number to get the lower range of your intensity scale.

Multiply your Heart Rate Reserve by .8 and add back your Resting Heart Rate to get your upper range of your intensity scale. Now you have lower and upper ends of the scale.

It may sound complicated, but it's simple. For example, let's look at a 50-year-old with a Resting Heart Rate of 70.

> 220 – 50 (age) = 170 Maximum Heart Rate
>
> 170 – 70 (Resting Heart Rate) = 100 (Heart Rate Reserve)
>
> 100 x .6 = 60 + 70 (Resting Heart Rate) = 130. This is the lower end of his intensity scale.
>
> 100 x .8 = 80 + 70 (Resting Heart Rate) = 150. This is the upper end of his intensity scale.

This person would need to exercise at a heart rate between 130 and 150 to benefit from exercising. (Keep in mind that blood pressure medication may impact your ability to elevate your heart rate to the rates suggested here. Always consult your physician before starting a workout regimen.)

The other method to determine intensity is qualitative. Qualitative basically means "subject to interpretation." The qualitative measure to gauge intensity is through a method called Rate of Perceived Exertion.

Imagine a scale of 1-10, with 1 being the absolute easiest activity requiring little effort on your part (sitting still, for example). At the other end of the scale, 10 is an all-out effort (running as hard as you can, for example). So 2 is still pretty easy and 9 is pretty hard.

Your Rate of Perceived Exertion should be between 6 and 8 — somewhat hard. Because this is your own perceived exertion rate, some individuals will differ based on exercise experience and capabilities.

TAKEAWAY: Training harder is not necessarily training better; training easy will not get you to your goal.

Warm up and Cool Down

Exercise is done against one's wishes and
maintained only because the alternative is worse.

~ George Sheehan

A muscle is like a car. If you want it to run well early
in the morning, you have to warm it up.

~ Florence Griffith Joyner

One of the most important components of an exercise session is a proper warm up and cool down. Both of these will work together to provide you with a safe, effective, and fun exercise session.

A warm up is designed to prepare the body physically and psychologically for the task or activity ahead.

As its name suggests, a warm up increases the temperature of the working muscles. Increased temperature will cause dilation of the blood vessels, which means they will widen and be able to move more blood to the working muscles.

Warm ups are generally divided into three basic types: passive, general, and specific.

A passive warm up increases the temperature of the working muscles without movement. While on the surface this may seem difficult, it's quite easily accomplished in a couple of ways.

Just putting on extra layers of clothing to increase body warmth is an effective method of increasing body temperature.

Perhaps you might sit in a sauna for a few minutes to increase your body temperature.

The use of analgesic balms and heating pads is also an effective way to locally heat up the working muscles.

A general warm up is designed to increase systemic circulation. Systemic means "system-wide." In this case, your body is the system, so to increase systemic circulation you would need to do some type of activity using oxygen and large muscle groups.

Walking and light jogging are both excellent methods of increasing circulation throughout the body. If you are inside, you could engage in a general warm up by riding a stationary bicycle or using an elliptical machine for several minutes.

While there is no set time for this phase, it should be noted that the shorter the event you are about to perform, the longer the warm up needs to be. For example, sprinters need to warm up a lot because they will go from resting to peak capacity instantly. Muscles have a tendency to pull if not properly warmed up.

Finally, a specific warm up would be doing the activity you're about to perform, but at a lower intensity.

For example, baseball players might simply have a catch before their game. About to go lift weights? Start light at first to give those muscles a chance to get ready for the heavy lifting. Going to do the elliptical for your workout today? Start slowly. In this case, you have combined the general and specific warm up into your activity for the day.

A cool down is most important when performing cardiovascular exercise.

Spend as much time on your cool down as you did warming up. It's recommended not to stop your exercise abruptly, as this increases pooling of deoxygenated blood in the system and can be harmful. Gradually reduce the intensity of your exercise session.

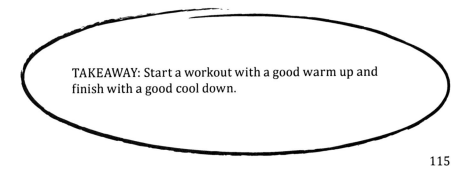

TAKEAWAY: Start a workout with a good warm up and finish with a good cool down.

In His Own Words:
Pete Rises to the Challenge

He who has a why to live for can bear
almost any how.

~ Friedrich Nietzsche

Your purpose in life is to find your purpose
and give your whole heart and soul to it.

~ Gautama Buddha

When I first joined the department, as a clerk in 1991, I weighed 250 lbs. and had never worked out in my life. I joined as a clerk because my fitness level was too poor to be a law enforcement or corrections officer.

At that time, you had to be able to bench press your weight and run 1.5 miles in a certain amount of time, neither of which I could do. Being 24 and full of energy and confidence, I joined a group of helpful officers who got me into good enough shape to pass the test at 225 lbs.

Twenty-three years later, in 2014, I found myself not quite so motivated. Stress and working a desk had taken their toll. I was once again 250 lbs., only now lacking the vigor of youth. I was in a rut.

I suffered from depression and hypertension. I had been diagnosed with heart disease and was taking testosterone, ED medication, cholesterol, and triglyceride medication. And my knees were killing me.

My doctor told me I would likely have a heart attack within ten years. I was 47.

Then I met Joe Serio and heard some of the things outlined in this book. Fortunately, some core ideas stuck in my mind. Above all, I came to realize that I'm the only one responsible for my happiness and that I can accomplish anything I decide to accomplish.

Eight months later, I weighed 210 lbs. The knee pain went away and my cardiologist was now saying I was his best patient. I no longer needed to take ED medication and took half the testosterone. I took the minimum amounts of cholesterol and triglyceride medication, and that's due to my genes.

The doctor said I was doing the best I can with the cards I was dealt.

Here's the plan I followed:

I exercised every day before I did any of the sedentary things I like to do. I didn't eat out on duty; I brought healthy foods that I enjoyed eating. I gave myself a free day to eat whatever I wanted, and I didn't beat myself up over any lapse, knowing that the next day would be better. I got on myself if I chose to have consecutive bad days.

I found activities and exercises I liked to do: walk the dog, bike, play football with my son, kayak, and walk around the neighborhood with my family. I examined how much time I watched TV or played video games, and realized that TV and video games had become my priorities.

Since then, I decided that 210 lbs. was too light for a guy of my height (6'7") and still effectively wrestle with the bad guys. I pushed myself up to 220 lbs. I now weigh what I want to weigh because of my own determination, not out of fear or lousy habits.

I still struggle from time to time. Sometimes I put on a few extra pounds and my body and knees remind me of it.

I have to tell myself that I'm the only one responsible for my life and that I can do whatever I choose to do. That puts me back on the path.

TAKEAWAY: Turning around your situation is possible. It's up to you.

Part 8

The Right Stuff

Lesson 48

Vince Lombardi and Fitness

Winning isn't everything — but wanting to win is.

~ Vince Lombardi

The greatest accomplishment is not in never falling,
but in rising again after you fall.

~ Vince Lombardi

Growing up in Wisconsin conditioned Matt to understand that his world revolved around one thing: the Green Bay Packers. He has vivid memories tossing the pigskin around with his father. The game would end abruptly with his father's comment, "The Packers are on."

Besides tremendous players, a couple of Super Bowl victories, and a rapidly-growing fan base, the Packers had Vince Lombardi, arguably the best head coach in football history.

Besides being a great coach, Lombardi was a great motivator. His players recount not only how he motivated them to be their best, but also to come together as a team to achieve their goal of winning.

Many famous quotes are attributed to Lombardi, and his words have meaning for those of us trying to improve our quality of life. Here are just a few:

"A man is as great as he wants to be. If you believe in yourself and have the courage, the determination, the dedication, the competitive drive, and if you are willing to sacrifice the little things in life and pay the price for the things that are worthwhile, it can be done."

Self-doubt and self-denial can prevent you from moving forward. Belief in yourself is the key to all of your success. You must develop that belief and have the determination to work toward achieving your goals. But it doesn't come without some sacrifice, whether it's money, time, or energy.

"Perfection is what we strive for — however, no one is perfect. But in the quest to chase perfection, we will catch excellence."

Chasing something that is important to you is a worthwhile venture. Working towards a goal of perfect fitness? There is no such thing. But if you set ambitious goals and are committed to them, you can have better fitness than you ever thought possible.

"Practice does not make perfect. Only perfect practice makes perfect."

You already know no one is perfect, but this quote puts into perspective that practice alone will not make you better. You need to do it right. When you practice with bad form, bad technique, and bad habits, you get worse instead of better. You know that from your experience in the academy and on the streets.

"Once you learn to quit, it becomes a habit."

This is one of the underlying reasons most people don't reach their exercise, fitness, and health goals. How many times have you begun an exercise program or started a diet only to give up after a short time? When you quit exercising once, it's fairly easy to justify stopping your program again...and again...and again.

"The difference between a successful person and others is not a lack of strength, not a lack of knowledge, but rather a lack of will."

Success is often said to be achieved when preparation meets opportunity. Opportunities arise every day. But the preparation for these opportunities takes willpower to persevere through all the obstacles in your way. Exercise is similar to that in many ways. There are a lot of reasons not to work out, and you have to have compelling reasons to want it badly enough.

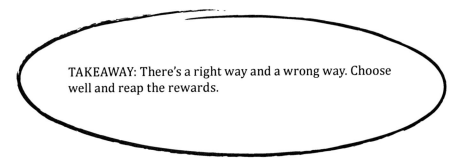

TAKEAWAY: There's a right way and a wrong way. Choose well and reap the rewards.

The Impact You Can Make

*A life is not important except in the impact
it has on other lives.*

~ Jackie Robinson

*You are here to make a difference,
to either improve the world or worsen it.
And whether or not you consciously choose to,
you will accomplish one or the other.*

~ Richelle E. Goodrich

You may be saying, "I'm no Vince Lombardi."

Well, maybe you are in some way.

One major reason law-enforcement officers should stay in shape is to strengthen their influence on people in the community, especially young people. You can be a leader like Vince Lombardi and help those around you strive for excellence.

As we all know, society has changed significantly over the past few decades. It used to be that, in many families, dad worked and mom stayed home all day.

If you're old enough to remember those days, then you remember having supervision, someone who was cooking meals regularly or preparing healthy snacks for you.

You probably had siblings or neighborhood friends you ran around with.

There were paper routes, shoveling snow, raking leaves, and all kinds of other part-time jobs to be done.

In school, you had at least one recess period and Physical Education classes. This kept you active and was helpful in releasing stress, getting oxygen to your brain, and assisted you in the learning process.

After school, you might have run home and then played "until the street lights came on." You would find things to do, places to explore, and make up your own games. You could ride your bikes to the park or play on the playground.

You were very active.

Over time, there's been a whole series of interrelated changes that has resulted in far less activity among young people: broken families, a decline in public nutrition, childhood obesity, slashed school budgets, and the rising tide of technology in every aspect of life.

What is the impact of this trend on law enforcement?

If the parents are not home after work, this leads to potentially unsupervised time. If kids have more idle time, they look for different things to do. Because just riding around and playing outside is now "dangerous," they may seek alternative activities.

Did you see the video of the police officer stopping his patrol car and throwing a football around with a little boy? Not only did that kid get a little bit of activity (as well as the officer!), this young man may have come away from that encounter with a whole different perspective of law enforcement.

The imprint of the importance of fitness in individual lives should be made at an early age. Police officers can act as role models in many ways throughout their careers, and perhaps one very important way would be to model fitness for impressionable minds.

TAKEAWAY: You are constantly making an impact. You get to decide if it will be positive or negative.

Jerard's Amazing Transformation

The triumph can't be had without the struggle.

~ Wilma Rudolph

A dream will always triumph over reality, once it is given the chance.

~ Stanislaw Lem

Jerard had a pretty typical childhood. He grew up playing sports and staying active. High school consisted of football, track, and powerlifting. After high school, he started focusing on lifting weights. His body weight increased to 250 lbs., but he remained lean at about 12% fat. This was a fit individual!

And then he went to college. For Jerard, his athletic career was seemingly over. There was no chance to play college football or run track. With those days behind him, Jerard embraced the stereotypical college lifestyle of fast food and alcohol. He would drink 64-ounce sodas and order 2 or 3 full meals at the local fast food place at one sitting.

Evenings were spent drinking multiple adult beverages. And with a significantly decreased activity level, his body weight quickly grew from 250 lbs. to 355 lbs. His body fat level increased from 12% to 38%. He was no longer a fit individual.

After graduating from college, he decided he wanted to get more active, but he sorely lacked motivation. The turning point came one day when he was on the couch and he dropped his phone on the floor. He tried to reach it but he couldn't get past his own girth. He had to drop to his hands and knees to get his phone.

Now he began to get active. He asked his roommate about a gym membership. He completely stopped drinking alcohol and cut out all processed foods.

In the first month, he lost 50 lbs. on one cardio session per week and four weight-training sessions. He attributes most of his weight loss to his lifestyle change: he ate "clean," meaning lots of vegetables and lean meats. He drank only water.

His day was planned around his workouts and his meals. He prepared all his meals in advance, laying out what he needed for 4-6 meals per day. He maintained this strict schedule for three years.

His weight went from 355 lbs. at 36% body fat to 225 lbs. at 9% body fat. He became a personal trainer at a health club and was instrumental in helping members achieve the success that he did.

A career in law enforcement had always been in the back of his mind. At 355 lbs. it wasn't a realistic option, but now he knew he could do it.

At the police academy, Jerard was one of the largest recruits. He went from not running at all to running 3-6 miles per day.

Jerard knew that until you put on the uniform and wear it for 12 hours a day, you don't realize how difficult it really is. From carrying around all the extra gear to your limited range of motion, the benefits to law enforcement of adequate fitness levels cannot be underestimated.

The questions that still drive him during his workouts include: Am I physically fit enough to handle any situation that I may encounter? Even though 90% of my time is spent sitting, am I prepared to deal with any situation in that other 10% of my day?

There is still a lot of peer pressure in his department to eat fast food and drink. Jerard has made the decision that his fitness level is more important than giving in to outside pressures.

TAKEAWAY: You got this! One step at a time, doing what you're supposed to do, will lead to success.

The Road Ahead

In three words I can sum up everything I've learned about life: it goes on.

~ Robert Frost

It is better to be hated for what you are than to be loved for what you are not.

~ Andre Gide

Now that you've finished reading this book, the road ahead begins with some basic questions you can ask yourself: Do I want to feel better? Do I want to look better? Do I want to have better relationships? Do I want my work to be more rewarding? Do I want to have a healthier outlook on my life?

Yes, all of these things are possible – for you!

Maybe you're at a point where you don't believe it. That's understandable, especially if you've been locked in the same mindset for many years. It becomes difficult to imagine that things can be different. It becomes difficult to imagine that you can be successful.

There are just two things you have to know:

1. Success is a head game. It's psychological. It only requires that you allow yourself to do something you've never done before. What you've been doing so far hasn't been working well, so what do you have to lose by trying something new?

2. If you burn more calories than you take in, you will lose weight. If you begin a weight-training program, you will grow muscle. If you stretch regularly, you will become more flexible.

One thing to keep in mind: you're not alone. Office Smith, Lee Stephenson, Pete, and Jerard were in your same position. Once they came to understand the two things listed above and answered "yes" to the questions at the beginning of this lesson, they improved their fitness and health dramatically.

They changed their lives.

And you can change yours, too. While sometimes it may not seem it, the power lies in your hands.

Getting fit and getting healthy is no different than any other pursuit: you have to believe you can do it, put a workable system in place, and go do it.

Remember that the people who get everything they want are not infallible. In fact, they have their fears just like you and me, but they don't make excuses. Even when the task is difficult or scary, they do it anyway.

And successful people don't beat themselves up when they fall off the wagon. You will stumble; you're human. It's part of the game. Get off your own back and get back on the wagon as quickly as possible.

I challenge you to visualize yourself having the fitness and health you want. I challenge you to put a plan in place to transform your life. I challenge you to then start living that plan. Start slowly, one day at a time, and success will come your way.

I would love to hear about your success. You can reach me at drjoe@joeserio. com.

The Takeaways

Lesson 1   If John can do it, why not you?

Lesson 2   Your body is one of your most important pieces of equipment. Prepare it the best you can.

Lesson 3   Exercise leads to fitness which improves your overall health.

Lesson 4   A combination of exercise and activity is the best approach for maintaining fitness and health.

Lesson 5   Exercise helps to reduce physical as well as emotional and psychological stress.

Lesson 6   Be aware of your own situation and the potential risks of exercise.

Lesson 7   Fear may be keeping you from having the health and fitness you want and deserve.

Lesson 8   Understanding your fears and feelings about your health is key to making lasting changes.

Lesson 9   Your excuses for not exercising are keeping you from getting what you need and want.

Lesson 10   You can change your belief about what you can handle.

Lesson 11   Don't wait for disaster to strike before preparing for it.

Lesson 12   Your belief in yourself and the task before you is critical to your success.

Lesson 13   Clear priorities will minimize distractions and keep you on the road to success.

Lesson 14   We create twice, first in our minds and then in reality. See your future and then go get it.

Lesson 15   No exercise strategies will matter until you decide and commit to succeed.

Lesson 16   Be SMART. Don't fool yourself into thinking that you have real goals if you don't.

Lesson 17   Don't worry if things don't go exactly as planned. Re-evaluate, stay flexible, and make changes.

Lesson 18   Set yourself up for success by getting rid of temptations and enlisting support from your friends or family.

Lesson 19   Put a system in place that streamlines your process to reach your goals.

Lesson 20   With a detailed blueprint in place, it becomes easier to reach your goals.

Lesson 21   Put all the pieces together to create a healthier lifestyle.

Lesson 22   Combine the information in this book for a multi-pronged approach to fitness and health.

Lesson 23   Let the five components work together to give you great fitness.

Lesson 24   Your cardiovascular fitness is the key to good health.

Lesson 25   Be sure to include muscle-strengthening exercises in your workout.

Lesson 26   Muscle endurance will help increase stamina and improve job performance.

Lesson 27   Stretching can strengthen your body and help prevent injury.

Lesson 28   You can change your body composition through a balance of exercise and nutrition.

Lesson 29   Your heart and lungs need to work together in order to deliver optimal performance.

Lesson 30   Reduce your belly, stretch, and stay active to decrease the likelihood of lower back pain.

Lesson 31   Choose the modality that's most enjoyable to you so you'll keep exercising.

Lesson 32   Without proper form and intensity, you will just be wasting your time in the weight room.

Lesson 33   Allow the large muscle groups to have a positive effect on the rest of the body.

Lesson 34   Various exercise opportunities exist. Find the ones that will benefit you the most.

Lesson 35   A "diet" lifestyle will add pounds to your waist; a nutritious lifestyle will help you keep fit.

Lesson 36   Use simple techniques to bring your portion size under control.

Lesson 37   Your body is about 60 percent water. You need to keep it that way!

Lesson 38   Vitamins and supplements can enhance body performance when taken correctly.

Lesson 39   Increase your activity and start moving gradually to an exercise program.

Lesson 40   Know what you're trying to accomplish and start slowly. Being safe is critical in an exercise program.

Lesson 41   Focus on the task at hand and perform the exercises in the correct way for best results.

Lesson 42   Fun is a critical ingredient in your exercise program.

Lesson 43   Forget about pain and choose discomfort. That's when you'll see great progress.

Lesson 44   The number of times a week you exercise is directly related to the results you will achieve.

Lesson 45   Training harder is not necessarily training better; training easy will not get you to your goal.

Lesson 46   Start a workout with a good warm up and finish with a good cool down.

Lesson 47   Turning around your situation is possible. It's up to you.

Lesson 48   There's a right way and a wrong way. Choose well and reap the rewards.

Lesson 49   You are constantly making an impact. You get to decide if it will be positive or negative.

Lesson 50   You got this! One step at a time, doing what you're supposed to do, will lead to success.

Sample Plan to Get Started

Pre-Week 1

- Visit your physician to see if there is any reason you shouldn't exercise.
- Set some goals: What are you trying to accomplish?
- Gather your resources – books, personal trainers – and seek advice!
- Gather your gear: appropriate shoes, clothing for gym, outdoor clothing.
- Make a meal schedule: Plan your meals in advance!

Week 1

- Day One: Begin gradually and don't overdo it!
- Cardio: Begin with 3 minutes and add as necessary.
- Weights: One set of about 8 different exercises.
- Flexibility: Six light stretches after your workout.
- Two days of cardio and two days of weight training.
- Nutrition: Remember to drink water!
- Begin portion control: Watch those serving sizes!

Week 2

- Add 2-3 minutes of cardio per session.
- Attempt to do three days of cardio and three days of weights.
- Remember, slow and steady gets those results!
- Always stretch AFTER your workout.
- Nutrition: Read those labels and watch for hidden excessive calories.

Week 3

- 4 days of cardio, adding 2-3 minutes per session if possible.
- Work on getting your heart rate up a bit more; stay in that target zone!
- Stay with three days of weight training and alternate those lifting days.
- Remember to stay hydrated.

Week 4

- Now it's starting to become a habit!
- 4 days of cardio, three days of weights.
- Add a little weight if the exercises are getting easier.
- Stretch after your work out. Hold each stretch 10-15 seconds each!
- Bet you are feeling a bit different about now...

Keep in mind that if you don't have a gym nearby, you can generate resistance by using stretch bands and do various push-up types of exercises to work out your triceps and other body parts using chairs, tables, and other furniture around the house. Simply Google: "How to Use Furniture to Exercise."

Lee Stephenson: My Path

I joined a local fitness center and started out doing 30 minutes of combined cardio on the treadmill and elliptical. I kept adjusting speed and incline and built upon that for about a month, approximately 6 days a week.

I was on light duty at the PD so on my lunch break I would walk 15-20 minutes on the treadmill at work. I'd go to the gym right after work and just built it in to my day. I've found exercise to be a great stress reliever, and I looked forward to taking advantage of that each day.

After about six or seven weeks of strict cardio, I began lifting light weights, researched the web, and started using a web app (Fitness Trainer). I found various exercises for different body parts.

At this point, I was lifting three days a week and doing two to three days of cardio with one day of rest. After about a month of this, I began working with a personal trainer three days a week and I did cardio two days. The trainer put me through a thirty-minute workout each session consisting of high-intensity interval training exercises focusing on different body parts each day.

When faced with difficult days, I look for motivation within myself and from outside sources. I talk to myself about whatever issue I'm having at any given time and quickly identify the excuses I'm using to rationalize my negative behavior.

I have come quite a long way in changing my mindset.

Instead of being negative about fitness and feeling that everything is stacked up against me, I look at what I have accomplished so far and acknowledge that I have made so many positive changes. I also set a weekly goal of how many days I'm going to exercise and what I'm going to do each day. Having planned it out, I feel obligated to myself to do it.

The same goes with my nutrition. I plan and prep the lunches and snacks I take to work each day. Then I go to the store, cook the lunches and pack the snacks in baggies. That way, each morning all I have to do is grab them and go.

Also, I subscribe to several Facebook pages that post a lot of good fitness, health, and motivational information, like Cooking Light magazine, Prevention

Magazine, Diabetes Support (excellent motivational posters), and Fit Cops. Plus, I have support from friends on different pages and my challenge group.

I have had some struggles here and there along the way, but an e-mail I sent to Joe Serio to let him know how I was doing led to an offer I could not refuse. He told me about this book he and Matt Wagner were writing concerning exactly what I was going through and sent me the manuscript to review. All he asked for was my critique and thoughts in return. Wow, I thought, what do I have to lose?

I found the manuscript to be just what I needed at this most important time in my life. I truly had a desire to be healthier and now I had a game plan in front of me. The book helped me in the following areas:

It explained to me about my fears: fear of how others saw me, fear of starting and finishing my journey, fear of increased medical issues if I didn't make changes, and fear of success and handling setbacks.

I learned about creating and implementing a system to be successful and how to set and reach my goals.

I learned about the basics of exercise, the five components of fitness, and the modalities of exercise and the science behind them that would assist me in reaching my goals.

The best thing about this book is that it explained so many things I needed to hear and know in such a simple way that even I could understand them. My story is so similar to Officer Smith's (Lesson 1) it was a little eerie.

I've gone through a total transformation both mentally and physically that I could not have achieved without the help of *Fifty Lessons on Law Enforcement Fitness*. I truly owe a debt of gratitude to the authors for having blessed me with this material! I have completely changed my mindset concerning getting healthier. If you've read the book this far, it's now time to do yourself a favor and take action!

I had total support and encouragement from my fellow officers and command staff to get myself healthy. I kept them informed of what I was doing by talking with them and tracking my activities and results on my Facebook page. They all bought in to my journey and gave me great support, advice, and encouragement.

The bottom line is I feel so much better at work. I have fewer aches and pains in my back. I am able to wear my vest with no issues and I'm much more active. My relationships at home have improved and, most important, my belief about what's possible has changed dramatically.

Acknowledgements

I would like to express my appreciation to all of the men and women in law enforcement who put a great deal on the line every day to help keep us safe. If in some way this book allows them to do their job better, and have a happier and healthier life, then we have done our job.

— Matt Wagner

I would like to thank Matt Wagner for making this book possible. I was fortunate to meet him during my time at Sam Houston State University (SHSU). And thanks to both law enforcement and non-law enforcement pre-publication readers of the manuscript: Nancy Anne Amato, Matt Bell, Bill Burt, Mark Cwirko, Garrett Demilia, Edward Jackson, Gerald Kim, Jerry Kovar, Roxane Marek, Will Rutherford, Wafeeq Sabir, Fred Schaaf, Helene Segura, Frank Serio, Tammy Spencer, Kristin Spivey, Lee Stephenson, and Darius Trugman. We hope the material in this book will motivate you to take the necessary steps to get everything you deserve.

— Joe Serio

Also in the
Law Enforcement Development Series

Dispatcher Stress: 50 Lessons on Beating the Burnout

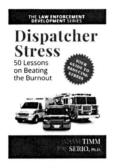

It's likely that you believe stress and burnout have to be part of your job as a dispatcher. If you could dramatically reduce your stress and improve your health, would you do it? What if you could:

- Feel relief from tension, frustration, and insomnia
- Relax in the midst of the toughest challenges
- Experience clarity and peace of mind again

Written by a former LAPD dispatcher, Dispatcher Stress: 50 Lessons on Beating the Burnout provides you with practical tools and techniques to change your thinking, your habits, and your stress right now. Learn to move past your exhaustion and anxiety.

Stop stress in its tracks, and have the career, relationships, and lifestyle you want!

ORDER NOW!

www.LEDtraining.com

Also in the
Law Enforcement Development Series

Leaving Blue:
50 Lessons on Retiring Well from Law Enforcement

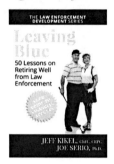

Does the thought of retiring from law enforcement make you nervous? Will there be enough money? Will you be able to do all of the things you want to do? Do you lie awake at night, weeks in advance of your event? Are you tired of living with the anxiety? Imagine turning all that around and feeling:

- Safe and secure
- Peaceful about money
- Excited about what you'll be able to do

In Leaving Blue: 50 Lessons on Retiring Well from Law Enforcement, Jeff Kikel and Dr. Joe Serio help you set yourself up for a retirement that's secure and enjoyable based on your top priorities, goals, and ambitions.

You've earned your retirement. Don't let your lack of preparation ruin it for you!

ORDER NOW!

www.LEDtraining.com

Also in the *Get the Nerve*™ *Series*

Time Management:
50 Lessons on Finding Time for What's Important

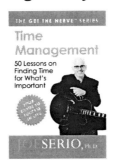

You often find yourself wondering where your time goes. Why aren't you getting done the things that are most important? Why aren't you making more progress in your career and life? Imagine having a system for turbocharging your time and feeling:

- More accomplished
- Satisfied
- Fulfilled

You can take control of your time, get organized, learn to say no more easily, and reduce the amount of stress in your life due to procrastination, perfectionism, and multitasking.

Don't let your bad time habits get in the way of your success!

ORDER NOW!

www.joeserio.com

Also in the *Get the Nerve™ Series*

Overcoming Fear:
50 Lessons on Being Bold and Living the Dream

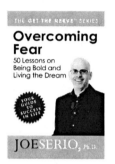

Take a good look at your life—is there something you would change if you could? Why is it that you don't already have whatever it is you're longing for?

- A successful career you enjoy
- Loving, peaceful relationships
- The time and money to do what you want

Whether you know it or not, chances are fear has become an obstacle in your path to reaching your goals. Until you learn how to move past it, you'll continue to be stuck.

Stop fear in its tracks, and Get the Nerve to have the career, relationships, and lifestyle you want!

ORDER NOW!

www.joeserio.com

Also in the *Get the Nerve™ Series*

Public Speaking:
50 Lessons on Presenting Without Losing Your Cool

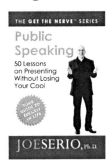

Does the thought of public speaking make you sick? Do you lie awake at night, weeks in advance of your event? Are you tired of living with the anxiety? Imagine turning all that around and feeling:

- Confident
- Calm
- Connected with your audience

Dr. Joe can help you manage your fear of public speaking so you can deliver killer presentations. In fact, as hard as it may be to believe, you can even learn to *enjoy* it.

Don't let your anxiety get in the way of your career!

ORDER NOW!

www.joeserio.com

About the Authors

Matthew Wagner, Ph.D., is associate Professor of Kinesiology at Sam Houston State University (SHSU) in Huntsville, TX. He received his Bachelor of Science in Criminal Justice from SHSU in 1980 and Ph.D. in Kinesiology from Texas A&M University in 1996. From 1980 to 2013, Matt was the owner of Nautilus Health Center in Huntsville. He served as a corporate fitness consultant from 2003-2009, developing and conducting fitness programs and testing for administration and line employees. He is co-author of Strength Training for Total Health and Wellness (2013) as well as Fundamentals of Weight Training (2011). He is a lecturer on fitness at the Law Enforcement Management Institute of Texas (LEMIT).

Joe Serio, Ph.D., is the founder of Law Enforcement Development Training (www.LEDtraining.com), specializing in personal leadership and individual responsibility and accountability programs for officers. He is also co-founder of The Healthy Dispatcher (www.thehealthydispatcher.com), providing wellness training to 9-1-1 dispatchers. He holds a doctorate in Criminal Justice with a specialization in Leadership and Organizational Behavior. Dr. Joe is a popular conference keynote speaker and trainer at police departments and other criminal justice agencies on leadership topics including positive interaction with difficult people, time management, stress reduction, customer service, managing personal finances, and others. He was the only American to work in the Organized Crime Control Department of the Soviet National Police and was Director of the Moscow office of the global corporate investigation and business intelligence firm, Kroll Associates. Dr. Joe is the author of the critically-acclaimed book, Investigating the Russian Mafia, as well as the founder of The Law Enforcement Development Series, which includes Getting Healthy: 50 Lessons on Fitness for Law Enforcement, Leaving Blue: 50 Lessons on Retiring Well from Law Enforcement, and Dispatcher Stress: 50 Lessons on Beating the Burnout.

CPSIA information can be obtained
at www.ICGtesting.com
Printed in the USA
FFOW03n1106160717
37840FF

9 780990 021650